Physical Therapy Musculoskeletal Examination:

The Clinician's Reference Manual

T0375266

First Edition

Any procedure or practice described in this book should be applied by the healthcare practitioner under appropriate supervision in accordance with professional standards of care used with regard to the unique circumstances that apply in each practice situation. Care has been taken to confirm the accuracy of information presented and to describe generally accepted practices. However, the author cannot accept any responsibility for errors or omissions or for any consequences from application of the information in this book and makes no warranty, express or implied, with respect to the contents of the book.

Order this book online at www.trafford.com
or email orders@trafford.com

Most Trafford titles are also available at major online book retailers.

Note for Librarians: A cataloguing record for this book is available from Library and Archives Canada at www.collectionscanada.ca/amicus/index-e.html

Printed in Victoria, BC, Canada.

ISBN: 9781-4120-6667-9

We at Trafford believe that it is the responsibility of us all, as both individuals and corporations, to make choices that are environmentally and socially sound. You, in turn, are supporting this responsible conduct each time you purchase a Trafford book, or make use of our publishing services. To find out how you are helping, please visit www.trafford.com/responsiblepublishing.html

Our mission is to efficiently provide the world's finest, most comprehensive book publishing service, enabling every author to experience success. To find out how to publish your book, your way, and have it available worldwide, visit us online at www.trafford.com

Trafford rev. 07/07/2009

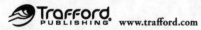 **Trafford** PUBLISHING® www.trafford.com

North America & international
toll-free: 1 888 232 4444 (USA & Canada)
phone: 250 383 6864 ♦ fax: 250 383 6804 ♦ email: info@trafford.com

Physical Therapy Musculoskeletal Examination:
The Clinician's Reference Manual

First Edition

Authored By:
Jonathan A. Di Lauri, MPT, CMP, TPI CGFI
Out-Patient Orthopedic Physical Therapist
Therapist and Owner of **JointCare Physical Therapy, LLC**
www.jointcarept.com

Content Editor:

Jeffrey DeBellis, MS, PT, OCS
Out-Patient Orthopedic Physical Therapist
Private Practice Owner

Style Editor:

Michael E. Goodman
Education Editor and Writer

Presentation Editors:

Viral Patel, SPT and Stephanie Roney, SPT
Student Physical Therapists

Special Thanks To:
~My wife Carmela for your continued support and understanding of my professional goals~
~My friends and family, especially Mom and Dad for giving me
the opportunity to dream and the talent to create~
~Chatham College Physical Therapy Staff (especially Pat, Raj, and Steve) and fellow classmates
for the knowledge and passion for what I do~

ABOUT THE BOOK

As students in graduate programs, we are aware of the overwhelming amounts of information we are expected to know and retain, not only for the national exam but also for the rest of our professional lives. While a student myself, I was constantly looking for condensed and easy-to-use reference material to help summarize these massive amounts of information. While studying for practical exams in orthopedic physical therapy at Chatham College in Pittsburgh, I condensed all my material (including my class and textbook notes) into a reference manual. This manual, in its early stages, was an invaluable tool for my classes, studying for my practical exams, and preparing for the national board exam. I continue to use the manual as a clinical reference and have shared it with student physical therapists and PTAs at our office. I firmly believe that this manual was the foundation for furthering my outpatient orthopedic physical therapy career.

Now I am sharing this manual to help you and other physical therapists increase your knowledge base and skills to enhance your work with your patients and support your future in the physical therapy profession. This book has received endorsements by members of the profession and those of the healthcare industry. (You can see some of these on the back cover of the book.)It is one of the most comprehensive yet inexpensive orthopedic evaluation tools on the market. I hope you will find it to be an invaluable addition to your professional library.

Physical Therapy Musculoskeletal Examination: The Clinician's Reference Manual is designed for: physical therapy students, physical therapists, physical therapist assistants, physical therapist assistant students, occupational therapists, occupational therapy students, athletic training students, athletic trainers, and any allied health professional looking to understand the vast skill of orthopedic examination. Whether you are trying to absorb massive amounts of orthopedic physical therapy information in school, studying for the boards, or already practicing, the outline formatted manual should help you better organize your clinical evaluation skills for all the major joints:

- Ankle
- Knee
- Hip
- Pelvis

- Lumbar Spine
- Cervical Spine
- Shoulder
- Elbow

This text includes:

- References from the most respected and widely used texts in physical therapy.
- Over 50 pictures of joint mobilizations and examination techniques.
- Simply laid out orthopedic examinations by joint and skill.
- Brief, easy to use, descriptions of manual muscle testing, goniometric landmarks, special tests, mobility testing (with photos), as well as components of taking a history.
- A built in notebook for you to create your own additions.
- End of chapter, blank examination forms to copy or to use as a template to create your own.
- An easy to reference content index and figure index.

ABOUT THE AUTHOR
Jonathan Di Lauri, MPT, CMP, TPI CGFI

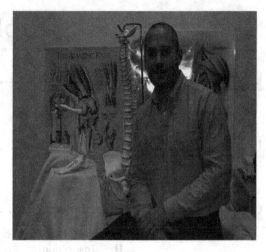

Jonathan graduated from Juniata College in 1997 with a degree in Holistic Allied Health (B.S.). In 1999, he earned his Masters Degree in Physical Therapy from Chatham College in Pittsburg, PA (MPT). Jon went on to earn his Personal Training Certification from the National Academy of Sports Medicine (NASM CPT) and his Certification as a Golf Fitness Instructor from the Titleist Performance Institute (TPI CGFI). In 2008, he became one of only 129 treating clinicians in the country to earn their manual therapy certification as a Certified Mulligan Practitioner (CMP). He has been approved as a CEU provider for the American Council on Exercise (ACE) and the National Strength and Conditioning Association (NSCA) and the National Academy of Sports Medicine (NASM).

Professional organizations of which he is a member include the Sports Medicine, Orthopedic, and Private Practice Sections of the APTA. He has observed multiple surgical interventions including: Shoulder Arthroscopy, ORIF of the Ankle and Hip, Open Rotator Cuff Repair, Sub-Acromial Decompression, Knee Arthroscopy, ACL Reconstruction, and Total Joint Replacement.

Jonathan Di Lauri has spoken publically in both community and institutional settings on a variety of topics related to Sports Medicine and Orthopedic Physical Therapy, research findings at the institutional level as well as one of the nationally featured speakers for the "Rehabilitation To Recreation" concept which he co-created.

Jonathan is currently the owner and physical therapist of JointCare Physical Therapy, LLC, an out-patient sports/orthopedic physical therapy practice in northern New Jersey. His clinical focus is based on accurate, thorough examination accompanied by individualized patient treatment plans including extensive patient education, therapeutic exercise, neuromuscular re-education, biomechanical taping, home exercise prescription, modalities and an emphasis on manual therapeutic intervention to return patients to optimal function.

In 2008, he launched a multidisciplinary Golf Performance Center combining the latest technology with the most effective interventions ever combined in one setting. Along with a foundation of Titleist Performance Institute Fitness Instruction, this experience includes: PGA golf professional lessons, physical therapy, personal training and fitness, Golf Simulation and use of the ATM2PRO Vertical treatment table.

His expertise is founded on manual, hands-on physical therapy with over 200 hours of continuing education, over 40 hours of orthopedic surgical observation, and 10 years of out-patient orthopedic experience focused on exceptional patient care.

Learn more about him and his practice at www.jointcarept.com

Table of Contents

Table of Contents

Table of Contents

Upper Quarter Screen
(By Skill)

I. Inspection

II. Active Motions with Overpressure (Assess end-Feel)
1. Active elevation of the shoulders (Arms overhead with palms together)
2. Active range of cervical spine (FB, BB, LSB, RSB, RR, LR)

III. Resisted Motions
1. Rotation of cervical spine (C1)
2. Elevation of the shoulder girdles, shrugs (C2, C3, C4)
3. Shoulder abduction (C5)
4. Elbow flexion and wrist extension (C6)
5. Elbow extension and wrist flexion (C7)
6. Thumb extension (C8)
7. Finger adduction (T1)

IV. Spring Test
1. T-7 and up (ROM, end - feel, pain)

V. Deep Tendon Reflex (DTR)
1. Biceps (C5, C6)
2. Brachioradialis (C5, C6)
3. Triceps (C7)

VI. TMJ

NOTES:

Lower Quarter Screen
(By Patient Position)

I. Standing: (Shoes and socks off)
1. Initial inspection
2. Active range of lumbar spine (FB, BB, LSB, RSB, RR, LR)
3. Heal walking (L4, L5)
4. Toe walking (S1, S2)

II. Sitting:
1. Rotation of the thoraco-lumbar spine (Add overpressure)
2. Patellar Reflex (L3, L4)

III. Supine:
1. Straight Leg Raise (Hamstring or Dural stretch) (Bilateral)
2. Long Sit Test
3. ROM of the hip (Flexion, IR, ER) (Bilateral)
4. Resisted hip flexion (L1, L2) (Bilateral)
5. Resisted knee extension (L1, L2, L3) (Bilateral)
6. Resisted ankle dorsiflexion (L4) (Bilateral)
7. Resisted ankle eversion (L5, S1) (Bilateral)
8. Resisted great toe extension (L4, L5)

IV. Prone:
1. Femoral Nerve Stretch
2. Ankle Reflex (S1)
3. Observe the gluteal mass
4. Spring Test from T7 down

CHAPTER I
ANKLE EXAMINATION

Ankle

NOTES:

I. HISTORY

1. Date of onset of symptoms
2. Mechanism of injury
3. Treatment to date for this injury
4. Diagnostic tests (X-Ray, MRI)
5. Current symptoms (Strength, range, edema, pain (0–10 Scale), immobility)
    A. Functional limitations
        a. Home
        b. Work
        c. ADLs
6. Medications not related / related to diagnosis
7. Past medical history
8. Work function
9. Patient's goals

II. INSPECTION

1. Size/shape/deformities (Involved side/uninvolved comparison may be necessary)
    A. Bony landmarks
    B. Girth-atrophy /swelling / color
    C. Calluses, corns, blisters
        <u>Hagland's Deformity</u>: (Pump bump)— Apex of the calcaneous
    D. Toe deformities
        <u>Hammer toe</u>: Hyperextended MTP, flexion of PIP, neutral DIP
        <u>Claw toe</u>: Hyperextended MTP, flexion of PIP and DIP
        <u>Mallet toe</u>: Only the DIP is hyperflexed secondary to a possible contracture
2. Varus / Valgus
    A. Knees
        a. <u>Knock Knee</u>: Genu valgus
        b. <u>Bowlegged</u>: Genu varus
        c. Medial / Lateral rotation of tibia / femur
    B. Heels
        a. <u>Subtalar Pronation</u>: Valgus
        b. <u>Subtalar Supination</u>: Varus
        c. <u>Equines</u>: Lacking dorsiflexion, congenital or acquired
    C. Forefoot
        a. <u>Forefoot Supinatus</u>: Acquired bony deformity, results in flatfooted medial arch
        b. <u>Forefoot varus</u>: Soft tissue deformity, pronation at the subtalar joint and inversion of the forefoot
        c. <u>Forefoot valgus</u>: (Congenital deformity) Supination at the subtalar and eversion of the forefoot when in subtalar neutral
3. Foot position
    A. Talar neutral

4. Gait
    A. Heel strike/ Ability to maintain the medial arch through mid-stance / Toe off

NOTES:

III. LOWER QUARTER SCREEN (See page 3.)

IV. RANGE OF MOTION [8]

1. Goniometry (Patient is sitting) (Assess end feel bilaterally)

    A. Ankle Plantarflexion: 0°– 50° / Dorsiflexion: 0°– 20°
        Stationary arm: Lined up with the fibular head
        Measuring arm: Lined up with the fifth metatarsal
            Apex: Lateral malleolus

    B. Foot Inversion: 0°– 30° / Eversion: 0°– 15°
        Stationary arm: Lined up with tibial tuberosity and shaft
        Measuring arm: Lined up with second metatarsal and toe
            Apex: Subtalar Joint / Dorsum of foot

    C. Subtalar Neutral: (Patient is standing in a natural position.)
        By palpating the head of the talus dorsally between the thumb and index finger at its medial and lateral aspects, the patient is asked to supinate or pronate the ankle until an even amount of the talus is felt at the thumb and index finger. The clinician notes the amount of motion required to attain neutral.

2. Active / Passive movement
    A. End feel
    B. Flexibility (Gastroc, Tibialis Anterior, Peroneals, etc.)
    C. Quality of movement

V. MANUAL MUSCLE TEST [7]

    A. ABductor Hallucis: (Patient performs great toe abduction against resistance.)
    B. ADductor Hallucis: (Patient performs great toe adduction against resistance.)
    C. Flexor Hallucis Longus: (Patient performs great toe flexion against resistance.)
    D. Extensor Hallucis Longus/Brevis: (Patient extends 1ST toe, resist flexion at DIP.)
    E. Flexor Digitorum Longus: (Patient performs toe flexion against resistance at DIPs.)
    F. Flexor Digitorum Brevis: (Patient performs toe flexion against resistance at PIPs.)
    G. Lumbricals: (Patient performs toe flexion at the MTP joint against resistance.)
    H. Peronei Longus/Brevis: (Patient performs plantarflexion and eversion against resistance.)
    I. Tibialis Posterior: (Patient performs plantarflexion and inversion against resistance.)
    J. Tibialis Anterior: (Patient performs dorsiflexion and inversion against resistance.)
    K. Soleus: (Patient performs bent knee heel raises, 20 repetitions.)
    L. Gastroc: (Patient performs straight knee heel raises, 20 repetitions.)

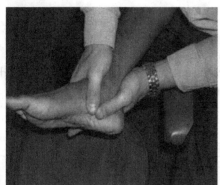

Figure 1

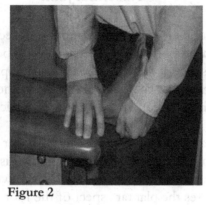

Figure 2

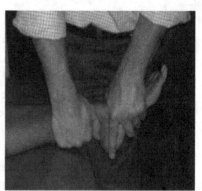

Figure 3

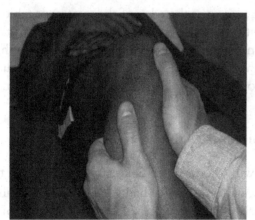

Figure 4

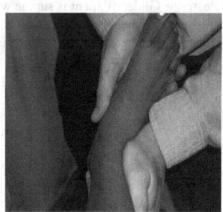

Figure 5

VI. MOBILITY TESTING [3] (Kaltenborn Method: 1=Hands on 2=Take up slack 3=Stretch)

(Accessory movements / End-feel of the involved and uninvolved sides)

Talocrural Joint

1. Distraction: (Patient is supine with the knee and hip flexed 90°.)
   (Figure 1) The clinician supports the leg between the elbow and ribcage. With the thumbs at the medial aspect of the foot, the clinician approximates the web space of one hand around the talus and the web space of the other hand around the calcaneous. The clinician's elbows are in at the sides. The clinician provides a distraction force.

2. Anterior Talar Glide: (Patient is supine with the foot over the edge of the treatment table.)
   (Figure 2) The clinician's proximal hand stabilizes the distal tibia just proximal to the malleoli, against the treatment table. The distal hand wraps under the calcaneous and the forearm presses the plantar aspect of the foot into slight plantarflexion. The clinician provides an anterior force with the distal hand. Posterior tibial movement may be substituted.

3. Posterior Glide: (Patient is supine with the foot over the edge of the treatment table.)
   (Figure 3) The clinician's proximal hand stabilizes the distal tibia just proximal to the malleoli. The web space of the distal hand wraps around the talus dorsally with the index finger pointed to ground and the remainder of the fingers wrapped around the dorsum of the foot. A posterior glide is performed. Tibial movement may be substituted.

Proximal Tibiofibular Joint

1. Antero-Posterior Glide: (Patient is supine with the foot on the treatment table and, the knee
   (Figure 4) flexed 90°.) Facing the patient, with the medial hand, the clinician stabilizes the tibia. With the lateral hand, the clinician grasps the proximal head and neck of the fibula using the thumb anteriorly and the index finger posteriorly. From this position, an anterior and posterior glide can be performed.

Distal Tibiofibular Joint

1. Antero-posterior Glide : (Patient is supine with the foot at the edge of the treatment table.)
   (Figure 5) The clinician posteriorly stabilizes the foot and ankle and approximates the medial malleolus with the lateral aspect of the thenar eminence to prevent it from gliding posteriorly during the mobility test (Not performed here in order to accentuate fibular glide) With the heel of the other hand at the anterior aspect of the lateral malleolus, a posterior force is applied. The positioning is reversed to test the medial malleolus.

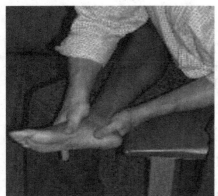
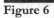

Figure 6

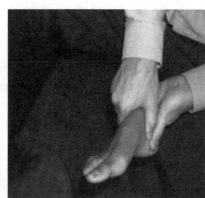

Figure 7

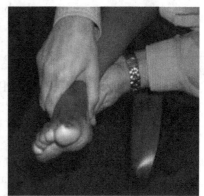

Figure 8

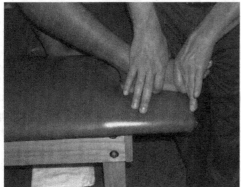

Figure 9

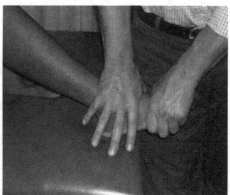

Figure 10

VI. MOBILITY TESTING (Continued)

Subtalar Joint

1. <u>Distraction</u>: (Patient is supine with the knee and hip flexed 90°.) The same technique as the
   (Figure 6) talocrural distraction is performed however, the dorsal hand approximates the navicular bone instead of the talus.

2. <u>Eversion Tilt</u>: (Patient is supine with the knee flexed 90°. The hip is flexed 90° and abducted.)
   (Figure 7) The clinician grasps the foot in the same manner as the distraction however both thumbs approximate the medial aspect of the calcaneous. The clinician performs **ulnar** deviation at the wrists and the thumbs force the calcaneous into internal rotation or foot eversion.

3. <u>Inversion Tilt</u>: (Patient is supine with the knee flexed 90°. The hip is flexed 90° and abducted.)
   (Figure 8) The clinician grasps the foot in the same manner as the eversion tilt however, both thumbs approximate just proximal to the medial aspect of the calcaneous and the fingers approximate the lateral calcaneous. The clinician performs **radial** deviation at the wrists and the finger pads force the calcaneous into external rotation or foot inversion.

Transverse Tarsal Joint

1. <u>Dorsal-Plantar Glide:</u> (Patient is supine with the knee flexed 60° and the heel on the table.)
   (Figure 9) With the proximal hand, the clinician fixes the talus and calcaneous to the treatment table with the thumb wrapping laterally and the fingers medially. The distal hand grasps the navicular bone between the thumb and web space dorsally. The fingers wrap around the foot. An anterior and posterior glide can be performed. The cuboid is tested in the same manner.

Naviculocuneiform Joint & Cuneiform-Metatarsal Joints

1. <u>Dorsal-Plantar Glide:</u> (Patient is supine with the knee flexed 60° and the heel on the table.)
   (Figure 10) Both mobility tests are performed the same as the transverse tarsal joint however for the NCJ, the proximal hand stabilizes the navicular bone and the distal hand mobilizes the cuneiforms. For the CMJ, the proximal hand stabilizes the cuneiforms, and the distal hand performs an anterior and posterior glide.

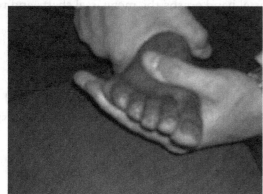

Figure 11A

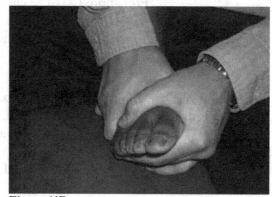

Figure 11B

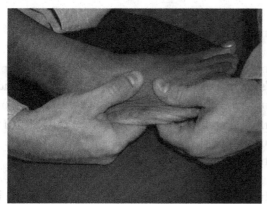

Figure 12

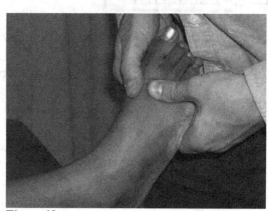

Figure 13

VI. MOBILITY TESTING (Continued)

Cuboid-Metatarsal Joints

1. <u>Rotation:</u> (Patient is supine with the knee flexed 60° and the heel on the table.)
   (Figure 11) With the proximal hand the clinician stabilizes the cuneiforms and cuboid.
   > Pronation: **(A)** The clinician's distal hand grasps the metatarsal shafts and rotates medially.
   > Supination: **(B)** The clinician's distal hand grasps the metatarsal shafts and rotates laterally.

2. <u>Dorsal-Plantar Glide:</u> (Patient is supine with the knee flexed 60° and the heel on the table.)
   (Figure 12) With the proximal hand, the clinician fixes the cuboid. The distal hand grasps the 4th and 5th metatarsals. An anterior and posterior glide can be performed.

Intermetatarsal and Tarsometatarsal Joints

1. <u>Dorsal-Plantar Glide:</u> (Patient is supine.) The clinician fixes one metatarsal shaft with the thumb
   (Figure 13) on the dorsal aspect of the foot and the fingers on the plantar aspect. The mobilizing hand grasps the adjacent metatarsal shaft in the same manner as the stabilizing hand and glides the shaft in a dorsal or plantar direction.

VII. SPECIAL TESTS [1]

1. Ligamentous Examination (Both involved and uninvolved side)

   A. <u>Anterior Drawer Test</u>: Tests the Anterior Talofibular Ligament. (Patient is supine with the foot relaxed.) The clinician's proximal hand stabilizes the distal tibia and fibula. With the proximal hand, the clinician secures the foot dorsally with the web space approximating the talus anteriorly. The clinician brings the foot into 20° of plantar flexion and draws the foot / talus anteriorly on the distal tibia and fibula.
      (+) Antero-lateral pain / hypermobility

   B. <u>Talar Tilt Test:</u> Tests the Calcaneofibular Ligament. (Patient is supine with the knee flexed 90°, the hip is flexed 90° and abducted.) The clinician supports the leg between the elbow and ribcage. With the thumbs at the medial aspect of the foot, the clinician approximates the web space of one hand around the talus and the other web space around the calcaneous. The clinician's elbows are in at the side. Both thumbs approximate the medial aspect of the talus. With the foot in the anatomical position (relaxed in plantarflexion), the clinician performs an adduction force to the talus.
      (+) Lateral pain / hypermobility

NOTES:

VII. SPECIAL TESTS (Continued)

1. Ligamentous Exam

  C. <u>Klieger's Test</u>:   Tests the Deltoid Ligament. (Patient is sitting at the edge of the table.) The clinician grasps the foot at the medial aspect of the great toe and provides an eversion force.
   (+) Medial ankle pain and hypermobility

  D. <u>Plantar Fascia</u>: With one hand, The clinician extends the toes and with the other hand, palpates the plantar aspect of the patient's foot.
   (+) Painful to palpation usually more proximal and slightly medial

2. <u>Morton's Test</u>: Tests for Mortons Neuroma caused by hypermobility or scar tissue at the nerve site. (Patient is supine.) The clinician grasps the foot and squeezes the 1st through 5th metatarsal heads together.
   a. Apply pressure at interspace between the metatarsals
   b. Apply pressure with a finger in the webs of toes

3. <u>Homan's Test</u>: Tests for thrombophlabitis /deep thrombosus. (Patient is prone, in ankle dorsiflexion.) The clinician squeezes the posterior crural compartment.
  (+) Hot to the touch and Painful (Refer this patient back to the M.D.!)

4. <u>Thompson's Test</u>: Tests the integrity of the achilles tendon. (Patient is prone)
  Same as the Homan's Test. The clinician wants to see plantar flexion of the ankle and any lateral/medial deviation.

5. <u>Burger's Test</u>: Tests the arterial blood flow to the foot and lower limb. (Patient is supine.)
  The patient's leg is lifted about 60° and held for 2–3 minutes while checking for blanching of the skin. The leg is then laid down in a dependent position and checked for color return.

6. <u>Tinel Test</u>: Tests the tibial nerve. The clinician taps the tibial nerve on the medial aspect of the malleolus.

7. <u>Tapping/Percussion</u>: Tests for fractures. The clinician's fingers are used to tap the foot including the malleoli and the tibial shaft.

NOTES:

VIII. PALPATION (Involved side)

1. Navicular bone
2. 1st metatarsal
3. 1st MTP, PIP, and DIP joints
4. Sesamoid bones, at the plantar aspect near the 1st MTP
5. 2nd – 5th MTP, PIP, and the DIP joints
6. 5th metatarsal and its head
7. Cuboid bone
8. Lateral middle and medial cuneiform bones (Palpate up the according metatarsal to find the joint between the metatarsal and cuneiform.)
9. Talus (Trochlea and head)
10. Calcaneous (Apex, middle tubercle, and sustantaculum tali)
11. Flexor Aponeurosis
12. Medial and Lateral Malleolus
13. Before leaving the foot, palpate the tendons:
    A. Peroneus Longus/Brevis
    B. Tibialis Anterior
    C. Tibialis Posterior
    D. Flexor Digitorum Longus
    E. Flexor Hallucis Longus
    F. Extensor Digitorum Longus
    G. Extensor Hallucis Longus
    H. Achilles Tendon
14. Tibial Crest
15. Tibio-Femoral Articulation (The grooves just below the patella)
16. Fibular Head
17. Take Pulses:
    A. Pedal Pulse (Dorsalis pedis, lateral to the extensor hallucis longus tendon)
    B. Tibial Pulse (Posterior to the medial malleolus with the flexor tendons)

IX. SHOE TYPES

1. Pertaining to the arch:
    A. Curve Lasted Shoe: Exaggerated medial arch
    B. Semi-Curve Lasted Shoe: Average medial arch
    C. Straight Lasted Shoe: Medial arch non-existent

2. Pertaining to flexibility:
    A. Board Lasted Shoe: No visible seams. Little flexibility.
    B. Combination Lasted Shoe: Visible forefoot seam. Forefoot flexibility / Rear foot stability
    C. Slip Lasted Shoe: Visible seams. Total flexibility throughout the shoe.

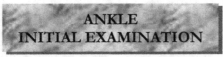

**ANKLE
INITIAL EXAMINATION**

HISTORY:

Patient Name: Date of IE: DX: R/L
Date of onset:
Pain: 0 1 2 3 4 5 6 7 8 9 10   Location:
Current symptoms:

Diagnostic Tests: Meds:

Functional Limitations:
Goals: PMH:

INSPECTION:

RANGE OF MOTION: * = PAIN

Plantarflexion: _____   Dorsiflexion: _____   Inversion: _____   Eversion: _____

MANUAL MUSCLE TEST: 0 – 5/5

ABductor Halucis: ADductor Halucis:

Flexor Hallucis Longus: Extensor Hallucis Longus/Brevis:

Flexor Digitorum Longus: Flexor Digitorum Brevis:

Peronei Longus/Brevis: Tibialis Anterior:

Tibialis Posterior: Soleus:

Gastrocnemius:

MOBILITY TEST: (+) = HYPOMOBILITY   WNL = WITHIN NORMAL LIMITS   (–) HYPERMOBILITY

Talocrural Joint   **Distal Tibiofibular Joint**   **Subtalar Joint**   **Transverse Tarsal Joint**
Distraction: Antero-posterior Glide   Distraction   Dorsal-Plantar Glide
Anterior Talar Glide: Eversion Tilt
Posterior Glide   Inversion Tilt

Proximal Tibiofibular Joint   **Cuboid-Metatarsal Joint**   **Naviculocuneiform**
Antero-Posterior Glide   Rotation   **Cuneiform-Metatarsal Joint**
                                       Dorsal-Plantar Glide   Dorsal-Plantar Glide

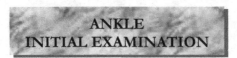

ANKLE
INITIAL EXAMINATION

SPECIAL TESTS: * = PAIN

Anterior Drawer Test:	(+)	(−)
Talar Tilt Test:	(+)	(−)
Klieger's Test:	(+)	(−)
Plantar Fascia:	(+)	(−)
Morton's Test:	(+)	(−)
Homan's Test:	(+)	(−)
Thompson's Test:	(+)	(−)
Burger's Test:	(+)	(−)
Tinel Test:	(+)	(−)
Tapping/Percussion:	(+)	(−)

PALPATION:

OTHER: (Girth)

ASSESSMENT:

GOALS:

Short Term (0–2 WEEKS)	Long Term (6–8 WEEKS)
1._____	1._____
2._____	2._____
3._____	3._____
4._____	4._____

PLAN: _____ x week for _____ weeks

_____   _____
SIGNATURE   LICENSE #

CHAPTER II
KNEE EXAMINATION

Knee

NOTES:

I. HISTORY [4]

1. Date of onset of symptoms
2. Mechanism of injury (Traumatic vs. Non-Traumatic)
3. Was the injury due to a traumatic event?
   > Yes: Possible ligament tear or meniscal tear
   > No: Overuse problem or degenerative condition
4. Was it a contact or non-contact injury?
   > Contact: Possible multiple ligamentous injury including: ACL, MCL, PCL, LCL or meniscus
   > Non-contact: Often ACL injury suspected
5. Did you feel a "pop" or a "click"?
   > Yes: Pops occur with ligamentous tears and meniscus tears.
6. How long did it take to swell up?
   > Within hours: Hemorrhage in the capsule (Intra-capsular)
   > Overnight: Synovial fluid build up (Extra-capsular)
7. Does the knee lock or buckle?
   > Lock: Often a meniscal tear flipping into and out of the joint

   Buckle: May be from quad weakness, trapped meniscus, ligamentous instability, or patellar
      dislocating.
8. Is climbing and descending stairs difficult?
   > Yes: Often patella-femoral problems
9. Are cutting maneuvers difficult?
   > Yes: Often ligamentous/meniscal injury
10. Is squatting (Deep knee bends) difficult?
    > Yes: Often meniscal tear or patella-femoral problem
11. Where is the type, severity and the location of the pain?
    > Medial joint line: Medial meniscal tear, medial compartment arthritis, medial collateral
    >   ligament
    > Medial tibia: Pes Anserine Bursitis
    > Lateral joint line: Lateral meniscal tear, lateral collateral ligament distal ITB, popliteus
    >   tendentious.
12. Diagnostic tests (X-Ray, MRI, Arthrogram)
13. Pain (Location, characteristics, intensity, at night)
14. Treatment to date for this injury
15. Current symptoms (Strength, range, edema, pain (0–10 Scale), immobility)
    A. Functional limitations
       a. Home
       b. Work
       c. ADLs
16. Medications not related / related to injury
17. Past medical history
18. Patient's goals

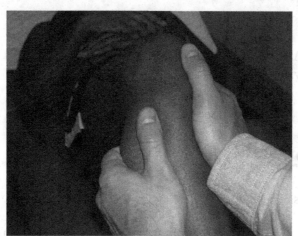

Figure 14

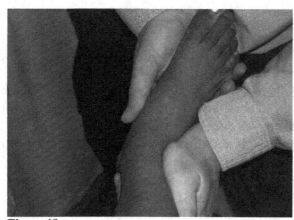

Figure 15

II. INSPECTION

1. Position of the knees (Tibial / Femoral Rotation)
2. Atrophy in the surrounding musculature
3. Swelling / effusion
4. Deformities
5. Valgus / Varus
6. Patellar Position (Alta or baha / sup or inf. / rotated or tilted)
7. Gait / assistive devices

III. LOWER QUARTER SCREEN (See page 3.)

IV. RANGE OF MOTION [8]

1. Goniometry (Assess end-feel)

 A. Extension / Flexion: (Patient is supine or prone, if tolerable.) 0°– 135°
 Stationary arm: Greater trochanter
 Movement arm: Lateral malleolus
 Apex: Lateral femoral condyle

V. MOBILITY TESTING [3]

Proximal Tibiofibular Joint

1. <u>Anterior-Posterior Glide</u>: (Patient is supine with the foot on the table and the knee flexed 90°.) **(Figure 14)** Facing the patient, with the medial hand, the clinician stabilizes the tibia. With the lateral hand, the clinician grasps the proximal head and neck of the fibula using the thumb anteriorly and the index finger posteriorly. From this position, an anterior and posterior glide can be performed.

Distal Tibiofibular Joint

1. <u>Antero-posterior Glide</u>: (Patient is supine with the foot at the edge of the treatment table.) **(Figure 15)** The clinician stabilizes the foot and ankle posteriorly and approximates the medial malleolus with the lateral aspect of the thenar eminence to prevent it from gliding posteriorly during the mobility test. (Not performed here in order to accentuate fibular glide.) With the heel of the other hand, at the anterior aspect of the lateral malleolus, a posterior force is applied. The positioning is reversed to test the medial malleolus.

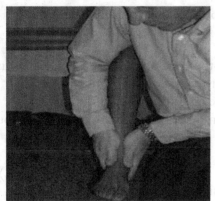
Figure 16

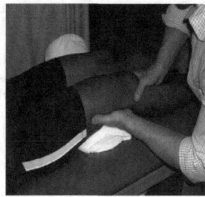
Figure 17

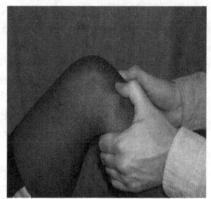
Figure 18

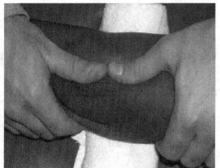
Figure 19A

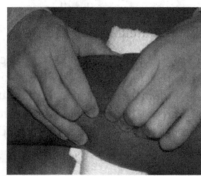
Figure 19B

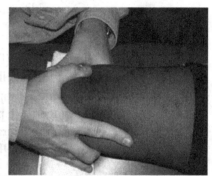
Figure 20A

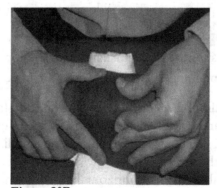
Figure 20B

V. MOBILITY TESTING (Continued)

Tibiofemoral Joint

1. <u>Distraction</u>: (Patient is seated.) The clinician grasps just above the malleoli with both hands. **(Figure 16)** A force is applied antero-inferiorly.

2. <u>Posterior Glide</u>: (Patient is supine with the joint line just off the edge of the table.) The clinician, **(Figure 17)** facing the medial aspect of the lower leg, grasps the malleoli. With the proximal hand, the clinician applies a posterior force to the anterior aspect of the proximal tibia, just distal to the joint line. A gentle traction force, with the distal hand, may be combined with this technique.

3. <u>Anterior Glide</u>: (Patient lies supine with the knee flexed 90°, same as the Anterior Drawer Test.) **(Figure 18)** The clinician stabilizes the distal leg by partially sitting on the patient's foot. The clinician places both thumbs anteriorly at the proximal edge of the tibial plateau so as to be able to palpate the mobility of the tibia when force is applied. The fingers of both hands wrap around the back of the proximal calf. The clinician leans back, providing an anterior force on the tibia.

Patellofemoral Joint

1. <u>Medial-Lateral Glide</u>: (Patient is supine.) The clinician places both thumbs over the lateral border **(Figure 19)** of the patella and the fingers over the medial aspect of the distal femur. The clinician applies a medial force through the thumbs.**(19A)** For the lateral glide, the fingers are placed over the medial border of the patella and the thumbs are secured on the lateral aspect of the distal femur. The clinician applies a lateral force with the fingers. **(19B)**

2. <u>Inferior / Superior Glide</u>: (Patient is supine and in slight flexion with a towel support) The **(Figure 20)** clinician secures the superior pole of the patella with the thumb and index finger and applies an inferior glide, parallel with the femur. **(20A)** With the webspace securing the inferior pole, a superior glide can be performed, parallel with the femur. **(20B)**

VI. FLEXIBILITY TESTING [1]

1. <u>Hamstrings</u>: (Patient is supine.) The clinician flexes the hip 90°, and the knee is extended. Always maintaining 90° of hip flexion, the knee flexion angle is measured.

2. <u>Ober's Test</u>: Tests the Iliotibial Band (Patient is sidelying, facing away from the clinician) With the distal hand, the clinician holds the knee in extension and the hip is fully extended. The clinician's proximal hand stabilizes the ilium and the patient's leg is lowered to the table.
   (+) Leg unable to reach horizontal / pain at the ITB

3. <u>Thomas Test</u>: Tests for hip flexor contracture. (Patient is supine at the end of the table.). The patient is instructed to hold the flexed knee and hip into the chest. The clinician lowers the other leg to the table. The clinician passively flexes the knee.
   (+) The leg is off the table with L/S extension
   (+) "J" Sign: Leg moves laterally 2° to ITB tightness

NOTES:

VII. MANUAL MUSCLE TEST [7] (Bilaterally)

1. <u>Quadriceps</u>: (Patient is seated.) A break test is performed in approximately 30° of flexion.

2. <u>Hamstrings</u>: (Patient is seated or prone.)A break test is performed at midrange.
   A. Biceps Femoris: External Tibial Rotation with a break test.
   B. Semitendonosis/ Semimembranosus: Internal Tibial Rotation with a break test.

3. <u>Gluteus Medius and Minimus</u>: (Patient is sidelying, facing away from the clinician) The upper leg is abducted and the patient resists a downward force.

4. <u>Hip Adductors</u>: (Patient same as above) The lower leg is raised to meet the abducted upper leg. The patient resists a downward force on the lower leg.

5. <u>Tensor Fascia Lata</u>: (Patient same as above) The patient's hips are slightly rotated toward the clinician. The patient's hip is slightly extended and abducted. The patient resists a downward force.

6. <u>Gluteus Maximus</u>: (Patient is prone with the knee flexed 90°.) A downward force is exerted on hip extension.

VIII. SPECIAL TESTS [1, 5]

1. **Cruciate Ligaments** (Clinician assesses the amount of translation and pain.)
   [Grading Scale: 0–5mm= 1[+] / 5–10mm= 2[+]/ 10–15mm= 3[+]/ 15–20mm= 4[+]]

ACL

A. <u>Anterior Drawer</u>: (Patient is hooklying with the knee flexed 90°.) The clinician sits on the patient's foot and attempts to anteriorly translate the tibia. The thumbs are placed anteriorly on the joint line. (Similar to the Anterior Tibiofemoral Glide described earlier)
   (+) Pain and hypermobility

B. <u>Lachman's Test</u>: (Patient is supine with the knee flexed 20° – 30°.) The clinician places his or her own knee under the femur of the patient, to maintain the angle and stability. The clinician's proximal hand stabilizes the femur with the heel of the hand and palpates the joint line using the thumb and index finger. The distal hand attempts to anteriorly translate the tibia. (Stresses the posterior capsule and the lateral band of the ACL)
   (+) Pain and hypermobility

NOTES:

VIII. **SPECIAL TESTS** (Continued)

PCL

C. <u>Posterior Drawer:</u> (Patient is supine.) The hand position is the same as for the Anterior Drawer, but the clinician attempts to posteriorly translate the tibia.
(The same positioning can also be used as described in the Posterior Tibiofemoral Glide)
(+) Pain and hypermobility

D. <u>Reverse Lachman's Test:</u> (Patient is supine.) The hand position is the same as the Lachman's Test but, the clinician attempts to posteriorly translate the tibia.

E. <u>Godfrey's Sag Sign:</u> (Patient is supine.) The hip and knee are passively flexed 90°. The clinician grasps the malleoli, lifts the test limb and looks for gravity to posteriorly translate the tibia causing a "sag" of the tibia posteriorly.

2. **Collateral Ligaments**

MCL

A. <u>Valgus Stress Test:</u> (Patient is supine.) The clinician holds the leg between the arm and the ribcage. With the medial hand, the clinician palpates the MCL. The clinician flexes the knee 10°– 20° and, with the other hand, applies a valgus stress to the joint.
(+) Pain and hypermobility

B. <u>Laterally Rotated Solcum Test:</u> (Patient is hooklying.) The clinician laterally rotates the tibia 15° and an anterior drawer test is done. (Tests the postero-medial capsule)

LCL

A. <u>Varus Stress Test:</u> (Patient is supine.) The clinician reverses the position from the Valgus Stress Test. The LCL is palpated, and a varus stress is applied.
(+) Pain and hypermobility

B. <u>Medially Rotated Solcum Test:</u> (Patient is hooklying.) The clinician medially rotates the tibia 30° and an anterior drawer test is done. (Tests the postero-lateral capsule)

NOTES:

VIII. SPECIAL TESTS (Continued)

3. Meniscus

A. <u>McMurray Test:</u> (Patient is supine with the hip flexed 45° and the knee flexed 90°.) With the proximal hand, the clinician palpates the medial and lateral joint line using the thumb and the index finger. With the distal hand, the clinician holds the foot and medially / laterally rotates the tibia.
    (+) Popping and pain.

B. <u>"Bounce Home" Test:</u> (Patient is supine.) The leg is held slightly above table at the calcaneous, with the knee flexed 20°. The knee is dropped into full extension.
    (+) Pain at the patella

4. Iliotibial Band

A. <u>Ober's Test:</u> This test was described in the Mobility / Flexibility section. (Page 29). It will be explained again, in its modified form, on this page.

B. <u>Noble Compression Test:</u> (Patient is supine.) The knee and hip are flexed, similar to a heel slide. The clinician applies pressure with the thumb, just proximal to the lateral femoral condyle. The patient is asked to extend the knee while compression by the thumb is maintained.
    (+) Pain at approximately 30° of knee flexion

5. Patella-Femoral Joint

A. <u>Modified Ober's Test:</u> Same as the Ober's Test previously described however, after the leg is lowered, the patient is instructed to actively extend the knee.
    (+) Pain over the lateral patella / femoral condyle

B. <u>Static/Dynamic Compression:</u> (Patient is supine.)
    <u>Static:</u> With one hand the clinician compresses the patella.
    <u>Dynamic:</u> The clinician places the thumb and index fingers on the superior aspect of the patella and stabilizes it while instructing the patient to contract the quadriceps.

C. <u>Apprehension Test:</u> (Patient is supine with 15° of knee flexion.) The clinician laterally glides the patella and observes the patient's reaction. The patient may also flex the quadriceps.
    (+) The patient is reluctant to contract the quadriceps in fear of patellar dislocation.

D. <u>Palpation of Odd Facet:</u> (Patient is supine.) The clinician moves the patella laterally as described in the patellar mobility section and the odd facet on the underside of the lateral patella is palpated.
    (+) Pain

NOTES:

VIII. SPECIAL TESTS (Continued)

E. Q-Angle / Functional Q-Angle: (Patient is supine.) The center of the patella is located and marked with a pen. Tibial tuberosity is located and marked. The ASIS is located and the patient is instructed to hold a finger on the structure.
    (+) Female > 18° / Male > 13°

    Stationary Arm: Mark on tibial tuberosity
    Apex: Mark on patella
    Movement Arm: ASIS

F. Lateral Pull Sign: (Patient is supine.) The clinician places the thumb of one hand on the superior border of the patella and the index finger of the hand on lateral border. The patient is instructed to contract quadriceps. The patella should move as much laterally as it does superiorly.
    (+) Lateral excursion is greater than superior excursion.

G. Crepitation: (Patient is seated.) The clinician places a hand over the patella and the patient extends the knee. The clinician feels and listens for crepitus. A stethoscope may be used to pinpoint specific locations of crepitus on the knee.

H. Patella Alta / Patella Baha: (Patient is seated.) The tibiofemoral joint line is palpated to gauge its relationship to the patella.
    Alta: Patella sits abnormally high, above the joint line
    Baha: Patella sits abnormally low, covering the joint line

6. Effusion Testing:

A. Brushing / Wave Sign: (Patient is supine.) The clinician starts the hand just below the joint line on the medial side of the patella, stroking proximally 2 – 3 times. With the other hand the clinician strokes down the lateral side of the patella.
    (+) A wave of fluid passes to the medial side of joint

B. Ballotable Patella: (Patient is supine.) The clinician applies the thumb and index finger lightly on both sides of the patella. With the other hand, the clinician brushes down on the suprapatellar pouch.
    (+) Separation of the thumb and index finger due to fluid.

C. Girth Measurements: With a tape measure, the clinician measures the girth of the knee bilaterally. Measurement locations should be properly documented and reproducible. (i.e. Joint Line, 5 – 15 cm up / down from the joint line)

NOTES:

IX. PALAPTION

1. Medial and Lateral Joint Line (Located at the inferior pole of the patella)

2. Hamstring Tendons

   Medial: Semimembranosus, Semitendinosus

   Lateral: Biceps Femoris

3. Quadriceps Tendon (Superior to the patella. The ligament is inferior to the patella)

4. Patellar (Odd) Facet (Depression on the underside of the lateral patella)

5. MCL (Crosses the joint line on the medial aspect of the knee)

6. LCL (Crosses the joint line on the lateral aspect of the knee)

7. Popliteus Region (Posterior aspect of the knee)

8. Gastrocnemius

9. Iliotibial Band (Patient lies supine and crosses one straight leg over the other.)

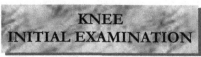

**KNEE
INITIAL EXAMINATION**

HISTORY:

Patient Name: Date of IE: DX: R/L

Date of onset:

Pain: 0 1 2 3 4 5 6 7 8 9 10   Location:

Current symptoms:

Diagnostic Tests: Meds:

Functional Limitations:

Goals: PMH:

INSPECTION:

RANGE OF MOTION * = PAIN

Extension - Flexion: _____

MANUAL MUSCLE TEST: 0 – 5/5

Quadriceps: Hamstrings:

Gluteus Medius/Minimus: Hip Adductors:

Tensor Fascia Lata: Gluteus Maximus:

MOBILITY TEST: (+) = HYPOMOBILITY   WNL = WITHIN NORMAL LIMITS   (−) = HYPERMOBILITY

Distal Tibiofibular Joint   **Tibiofemoral Joint**
Antero-posterior Glide   Distraction
Posterior Glide

Proximal Tibiofibular Joint   **Patellofemoral Joint**
Antero-Posterior Glide   Medial-Lateral Glide
                                            Inferior Glide

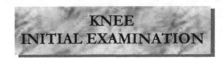

KNEE
INITIAL EXAMINATION

SPECIAL TESTS: * = PAIN

Collateral Ligaments

Laterally Rotated Solcum Test	(+)	(−)
Varus Stress Test:	(+)	(−)
Valgus Stress Test	(+)	(−)
Medially Rotated Solcum Test	(+)	(−)

Cruciate Ligaments

Godfrey's Sag Sign	(+)	(−)
Anterior Drawer	(+)	(−)
Posterior Drawer	(+)	(−)
Lachman's Test	(+)	(−)
Reverse Lachman's Test	(+)	(−)

Effusion Testing

Brushing / Wave Sign	(+)	(−)
Ballotable Patella	(+)	(−)

Meniscus

McMurray Test	(+)	(−)
"Bounce Home" Test	(+)	(−)

Patella-Femoral Joint

Modified Ober's Test	(+)	(−)
Static Compression	(+)	(−)
Apprehension Test	(+)	(−)
Lateral Pull Sign	(+)	(−)
Q –Angle	_____	

Iliotibial Band

Noble Compression Test	(+)	(−)
Ober's Test	(+)	(−)

PALPATION:

OTHER: (Girth)

ASSESSMENT:

GOALS:

Short Term (0 - 2 WEEKS)	Long Term (6–8 WEEKS)
1._____	1._____
2._____	2._____
3._____	3._____
4._____	4._____

PLAN: ____ x week for _____ weeks

_____   _____

SIGNATURE   **LICENSE #**

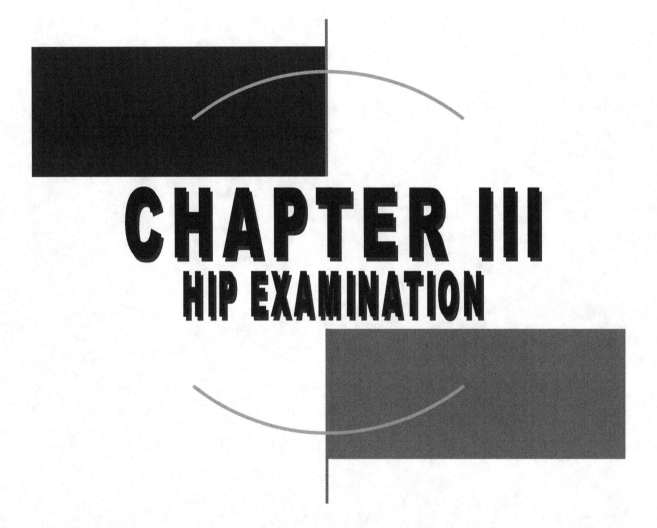

CHAPTER III
HIP EXAMINATION

NOTES:

I. HISTORY

1. Date of onset of symptoms
2. Mechanism of injury (Traumatic vs. Non-Traumatic)
3. Current symptoms (Strength, range, edema, pain immobility)
    A. Functional limitations
        a. Home
        b. Work
        c. ADLs
4. Diagnostic tests (X-Ray, MRI, and Arthrogram)
5. Pain (Location, characteristics, intensity, at night)
6. Medications related to injury
7. Treatment to date for this injury
8. Past medical history
9. Work function
10. Patient's goals

II. INSPECTION [5] (Anterior, Lateral, Posterior)

1. Position of the hip
    A. Anteversion: An increase in the angle of torsion
    B. Retroversion: A decrease in the angle of torsion
2. Atrophy
    A. Gluteal Mass
    B. Quadriceps
3. Swelling
4. Deformities
5. Valgus / Varus
6. Discoloration
7. Assistive devices
8. Gait
    A. Gluteal-Medial Lurch: (While on the affected limb) The patient presents with a lateral trunk lean due to ipsilateral hip abductor muscle weakness.
    B. Trendelenberg Gait: (While on the affected limb) The patient presents with an ipsilateral trunk lean and contralateral pelvic drop.

III. LOWER QUARTER SCREEN (See Page 3)

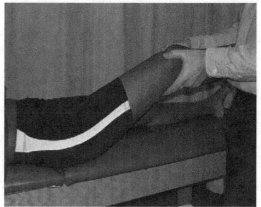

Figure 21

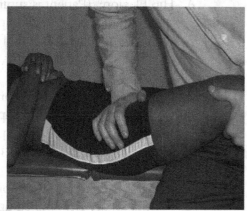

Figure 22

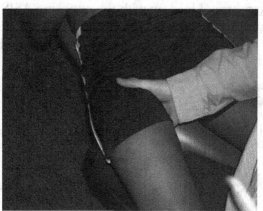

Figure 23

IV. RANGE OF MOTION [8]

1. Goniometry (Assess end-feel)

    A. <u>Hip Flexion:</u> (Patient is supine.) 0°–120°
        <u>Stationary arm:</u> Lined up even with the body
        <u>Movement arm:</u> Lateral femoral condyle
            <u>Apex:</u> Greater trochanter

    B. <u>Hip Extension:</u> (Patient is prone.) 0°–30°
        <u>Stationary arm:</u> Lined up even with the body
        <u>Movement arm:</u> Lined up with the lateral femoral condyle
            <u>Apex:</u> Greater trochanter

    C. Medial / Lateral Hip Rotation: (Patient is prone with the knees flexed 90°.) 0°– 45°
        <u>Stationary arm:</u> Lined up parallel to the table
        <u>Movement arm:</u> Lined up with the tibia
            <u>Apex:</u> Knee (Patella)

    D. Hip ABduction: 0° – 45° / ADduction: 0°– 30° (Patient is supine.)
        <u>Stationary arm:</u> Lined up with the opposing ASIS
        <u>Movement arm:</u> Lined up with the center of the femur
            <u>Apex:</u> ASIS of the joint being measured

V. FLEXIBILITTY TESTING

1. Hamstrings / Modified Ober's Test / Thomas Test / Ely's Test: (See page 29.)

VI. MOBILITY TESTING [3]

(Patient's hip should be in the open pack position of 30° of flexion, 30° abduction, and external rotation.)

1. <u>Inferior Glide:</u> (Patient is supine.) The clinician wraps both hands just proximal to the knee. **(Figure 21)** The clinician leans back and provides an infero-lateral force.

2. <u>Posterior Glide:</u> (Patient is supine.) With the distal arm, the leg is held in the open-pack **(Figure 22)** position. The proximal hand is placed at the proximal anterior thigh, and a posterior force is provided.

3. <u>Distraction:</u> (Patient is supine.) With the distal arm, the leg is held in the open-pack position. **(Figure 23)** The proximal hand is placed at the proximal, medial thigh, and a disto-lateral force parallel to the neck of the femur is applied.

NOTES:

VII. MANUAL MUSCLE TESTING[7]

1. Iliopsoas: (Patient is supine.) A straight leg raise is performed and pressure is applied against the femur.

2. Gluteus Medius / Minimus: (Patient is sidelying, away from the clinician.) The pelvis is neutral and the leg is abducted and extended. Pressure is applied toward the table.

3. TFL: (Patient is in the same position as above.) The leg is abducted and slightly flexed. Pressure is applied toward the table.

4. Hip Adductors: (Patient is in the same position as above.)The top leg is abducted and supported. The bottom leg is raised, and resistance is applied.

5. Hamstring: (Patient is prone with the knee flexed.) Resistance is applied against knee flexion.

6. Gluteus Maximus: (Patient is prone.) A straight leg raise is performed. Resistance is applied.

7. Hip Rotators: (Patient is seated.) Both internal and external rotation are performed. Lateral or medial resistance is applied along the tibia.

VIII. SPECIAL TESTS [1,5]

1. Patrick-Faber Test: Tests the articulation at the hip. (Patient is supine.) The patient places the leg in the figure 4 position. The clinician applies pressure to the bent knee.
   (+) Pain.

2. Scour Test: Tests postero-lateral capsule. (Patient is supine.) The hip is flexed to 90° and the knee is fully flexed. The clinician applies an axial load downward on the knee while moving through adduction, flexion, and medial rotation, followed by abduction and lateral rotation.
   (+) Pain.

3. Sign of the Buttock: Tests for space occupying lesion. (Patient is supine.) The extended hip is brought into flexion until resistance is met. The knee is then flexed.
   (+) Further hip flexion is absent when the knee is flexed.

4. Thomas Test: (See Page 29)

NOTES:

VIII. SPECIAL TESTS (Continued)

5. <u>Leg Length Tests</u>: The long sit test can be performed as in the lower quarter screen or the Weber-Barstow Maneuver is performed, and a measurement is taken.

(True) <u>Proximal end</u>:   **Iliac Crest**   **Greater Trochanter**   **Knee joint line**
to   to   to
<u>Distal end</u>: **Greater Trochanter**   **Lateral knee joint line**   **Medial malleolus**
(Coxa Vara/Valga)   (Femoral Shortening)   (Tibial Shortening)

(Apparent/functional) <u>Proximal end</u>: Belly button
<u>Distal end</u>: Medial malleoli

6. <u>Piriformis Test</u>: Tests the tightness of piriformis muscle. (Patient is prone.) The knees are flexed to 90° and brought together. Both femurs are then allowed to fall into medial rotation.
(+) One leg does not rotate as far as the other does.

7. <u>Trendelenburg's Test</u>: Tests hip abductors. (Patient is standing on the affected limb only.) The patient performs heel raises.
(+) Pelvis drops to the opposite side.

8. <u>Gluteus Medius Lurch</u>: Same test as the Trendelenburg Test.
(+) Trunk leans toward the affected limb.

IX. PALPATION

1. Iliac Crest
2. Greater Trochanter
3. ASIS
4. Tensor Fascia Lata
5. Femoral Triangle (Femoral Pulse)
    A. Sartorius
    B. Inguinal ligament
    C. Hip Adductor Musculature
6. ADductor Group
7. Hamstring Tendons
    A. Medial: Semimembranosus
              Semitendinosus
    B. Lateral: Biceps Femoris
8. PSIS

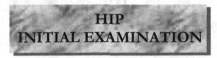

HIP
INITIAL EXAMINATION

HISTORY:

    Patient Name: Date of IE: DX: R/L

    Date of onset:

    Pain: 0 1 2 3 4 5 6 7 8 9 10   Location:

    Current symptoms:

    Diagnostic Tests: Meds:

    Functional Limitations:

    Goals: PMH:

INSPECTION:

RANGE OF MOTION: * = PAIN

Flexion: _____   Extension: _____   Abduction: _____   IR: _____   ER: _____

MANUAL MUSCLE TEST: 0 – 5/5

    Quadriceps: Hamstrings:

    Gluteus Medius/Minimus: Hip Adductors:

    Tensor Fascia Lata: Gluteus Maximus:

    Hip Medial Rotation: Hip Lateral Rotation:

    Iliopsoas:

MOBILITY TEST: (+) = HYPOMOBILITY   **WNL** = WITHIN NORMAL LIMITS   **(–)** = HYPERMOBILITY

        Femoral – Acetabular Joint

        Distraction

        Posterior Glide

        Inferior Glide

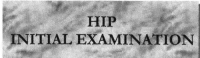

**HIP
INITIAL EXAMINATION**

SPECIAL TESTS: * = PAIN

Modified Ober's Test:	(+)	(–)
Ober's Test:	(+)	(–)
Scour Test:	(+)	(–)
Patrick-FABER Test:	(+)	(–)
Sign of the Buttock:	(+)	(–)
Thomas Test:	(+)	(–)
Piriformis Test:	(+)	(–)
Trendelenberg Test:	(+)	(–)
Gluteus Medius Lurch:	(+)	(–)
Leg Length Test:	(+)	(–)

		LEFT	RIGHT
(True)	1. Iliac Crest to Greater Trochanter	_____	_____
	2. Greater Trochanter to Lateral knee joint line	_____	_____
	3. Lateral Knee joint line to Medial malleolus	_____	_____
(Apparent/Functional)	1. Belly button to Medial malleolus	_____	_____

PALPATION:

OTHER:

ASSESSMENT:

GOALS:

Short Term (0–2 WEEKS)	Long Term (6–8 WEEKS)
1._____	1._____
2._____	2._____
3._____	3._____
4._____	4._____

PLAN: ____ x week for _____ weeks

_____   _____

SIGNATURE   LICENSE #

CHAPTER IV
PELVIC EXAMINATION

NOTES:

I. HISTORY

1. Date of onset of symptoms
2. Mechanism of injury (Traumatic vs. Non-Traumatic)
3. Treatment to date for this injury
4. Current symptoms (Strength, range, edema, pain (0–10 Scale), immobility)
    A. Functional limitations
        a. Home
        b. Work
        c. ADLs

5. Pain (Location, LE radiculopathy, characteristics, intensity, nocturnal)
6. Medications related to injury
7. What makes the symptoms better or worse?
8. Loss of bowel or bladder control
9. Sleep disturbances
10. Diagnostic tests

    A. MRI: (Magnetic Resonance Imaging) Magnetic waves are used to take pictures of slices of the spine. Allows vision of soft tissue, bones, nerves, and disks.
    B. CAT Scan: (Computer Assisted Tomography) X-ray cross sectional views showing the bones of the spine, similar to an MRI.
    C. Myelogram: A test involving placing a dye that shows up on X-ray, into the spinal sac. Will show the places where there is spinal compression.
    D. Discogram: A test where dye is injected directly into the disk at an area of the nucleus pulposus. The dye injection may cause "the pain" or a CAT scan or X-ray will pick up a herniation.
    E. Electromyogram: Looks at the function of the nerve roots leaving the spine. Electrodes placed in the muscles of the lower extremity help identify abnormal nervous signals.
    F. Bone Scan: Helps locate the affected area of the spine. A radioactive chemical is injected into the bloodstream. The chemical attaches itself to areas of bone that are undergoing rapid change. These appear as dark areas on the film.

11. Past medical history
12. Work function
13. Patient's goals

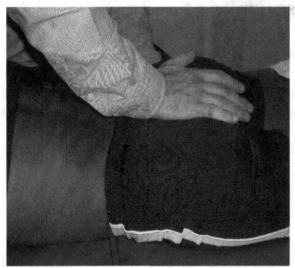

Figure 25

II. INSPECTION

1. Posture (Shift)
2. Atrophy (Standing behind the patient, the clinician looks at the back in extension and flexion)
3. Symmetry of bony landmarks (i.e. Iliac Crests, PSIS, ASIS, Spinous Processes)
4. Swelling
5. Deformities (Scoliosis)
6. Bracing
7. Ability to disrobe

III. LOWER QUARTER SCREEN (See page 3.)

IV. RANGE OF MOTION (Lumbar Active-Passive Movements)

Initial pain rating should be established in order to compare movements and pain intensities. Also, the clinician should be in a position to assess the segmental spinal movements. (Patient is standing.)

1. Flexion / Extension

2. Sidebending

3. Sidegliding / Translocation

4. Rotation

V. FLEXIBILITY TESTING

1. Hamstrings / Modified Ober's Test / Thomas Test / Ely's Test: (See page 29.)

VI. MOBILITY TESTING[3]

1. Posterior-Anterior Glides (Spring Test): (Patient is supine.) The clinician approximates the **(Figure 25)** sacrum with the ulnar border of the distal hand. The clinician applies an anterior force through proximal sacrum testing nutation (flexion) and through the distal sacrum testing counternutation (extension). A pad may be used to decrease the discomfort at the contact point. The clinician assesses: End feel, Muscle guarding, Symmetry, and Motion comparisons.

NOTES:

VII. MANUAL MUSCLE TESTING [7] (Modified)

1. Back Extensors: (Patient is prone with hands behind the head) The patient extends through full range.

    A. Grade: 5/5 – Full range and resistance
                4/5 – Same as above, the patient cannot maintain end-range
                3/5 – Completes range with the arms at the sides
                2/5 – Partial range
                1/5 – Palpable contraction

2. Abdominals (Rectus): (Patient is supine with hands behind the head) The patient curls up, clearing the scapula from the ground.

    A. Grade: 5/5 – Able to come to sitting position with back curled
                4/5 – Able to sit with the arms across the chest
                3/5 – Able to sit with the arms outstretched
                2/5 – Unable to complete full motion
                1/5 – Palpable contraction

3. Trunk Rotation(Obliques): (Patient is supine with hands behind the head) The patient sits up and simultaneously rotates the trunk.

    A. Grade: 5/5 – Full range and hold with hands behind head
                4/5 – Full range with the hands at the sides
                3/5 – Partial range with the hands at the side
                2/5 – Able to approximate the ileum and the ribs
                1/5 – Palpable contraction

Pelvis

NOTES:

VIII. SPECIAL TESTS [1,3]

1. <u>Straight Leg Raise</u> : Nerve tension test. (Patient is supine.) The leg is straightened and raised. Variations include asking the patient simultaneously to raise the head, dorsiflex the foot, and adduct the leg.

   (+) Nerve tension pain around 30° of the leg raise.

2. <u>Hoover Test</u>: Tests for malingering / Wadell Sign. (Patient is supine.) The clinician places one hand under each calcaneous and asks the patient to perform a SLR.

   (+) Clinician feels minimal to no downward force on the opposing foot.

3. <u>Sign of the Buttocks</u>: Tests for a space occupying lesion. (Patient is supine.) The clinician brings the leg into end range hip flexion. The clinician bends the knee to complete further possible range.

   (+) No further range after knee is flexed.

4. <u>Femoral Nerve Stretch</u>: Tests for lesions of the femoral nerve. (Patient is prone) The clinician places the proximal hand superior to the gluteal mass. With the caudal hand, the clinician flexes the knee 90° and extends the hip.

   (+) Provocation of nerve tension pain.

5. <u>Spring Test</u>: Provocation test at the spine. (Patient is prone.) The clinician applies a posterior to anterior mobilization to the lumbar vertebrae using the ulnar aspect of the hand against the spinous process of the vertebra being tested.

   (+) Provocation of the pain. Helps identify the level of involvement.

6. <u>Sorensen Test</u>: Tests lumbar paraspinals. (Patient is prone with trunk in neutral over the edge of table.) The patient is instructed to extend and hold for as long as possible.

   (+) Holding 1 minute or less. (Approximately 3 minutes is normal)

7. <u>Distraction Test</u>: Wadell Sign for the SLR. (Patient is seated.) The knee is brought into extension. (simulating the supine SLR) while the patient is distracted.

   (+) No pain (Patient should experience the same pain as with the SLR)

8. <u>Valsalva Maneuver</u>: Tests intrathecal pressure at the spine. (Patient is seated.) The patient is asked to hold breath and push, as if having a bowel movement.

   (+) Lower back and Sciatic pain.

NOTES:

VIII. SPECIAL TESTS (Continued)

9. <u>Sitting Flexion Test</u>: (Seated position eliminates the effects of the hamstrings.)

(The patient is seated away from the clinician with the knees flexed 90° resting on a chair.) The clinician maintains both thumbs on either PSIS. The patient is asked to bend forward.

(+) Asymmetrical movement of the PSIS indicates **SI** involvement. The side with more cranial motion reveals the side of hypermobility or hypomobility.

10. <u>Standing Flexion Test</u>: (Standing position involves the hamstrings) (Patient is standing.)

The clinician maintains thumb position on both PSIS. The patient is asked to bend forward.

(+) Asymmetrical movement of the PSIS indicates **IS** involvement. The side with more cranial motion reveals the side of hypermobility or hypomobility.

11. <u>Stork Test</u>: Tests for Pars interarticularis stress fracture / facet involvement.

(Patient stands on one leg) The patient is instructed to extend backwards.

(+) Pain on the ipsilateral side. (Rotation may be incorporated for facet involvement)

(+) Pain on the side of rotation.

12. <u>Iliac Compression Test</u>: Tests for sacroiliac involvement. (Patient is supine.) The clinician crosses his or her hands and places them on either ASIS. The clinician then forces the ileum apart.

(+) Pain at the iliosacral junction posteriorly (Sacroiliac Ligaments).

13. <u>Iliac Gapping Test</u>: Tests for Sacroiliac involvement. (Patient is sidelying.) The clinician pushes down on the iliac crest.

(+) Pain at the iliosacral junction posteriorly.

14. <u>Gillet's Test</u>: Tests for pelvic hypomobility. (Patient is standing.) The clinician maintains thumb position on both PSIS. The patient then brings one knee to chest. The PSIS on the flexed side should drop.

(+) PSIS of the flexing hip moves minimally or remains still.

Pelvis

NOTES:

IX. **PALPATION** (Symmetry between opposing landmarks)

1. Iliac crests
   Standing and sitting. Look for symmetry.

2. Ischial Tuberosity
   The clinician can find them when the patient is standing with the hip fully flexed or the patient seated / sidelying.

         a. Site of the hamstring origin.

3. Spinous Processes
   Between the iliac crests. Location of L-4

4. Transverse Processes
   On either side of the spinous process. The clinician palpates the ipsilateral process and compresses the contralateral side to feel movement posteriorly.

5. Sacral Sulcus
   Medial gap between the PSIS. Check for symmetrical depth.

6. Pubic Tubercles
   Instruct the patient to palpate the tubercles first. Then, place the hands over the patient's and check for height / pubic symphysis, and anterior / posterior displacement.

7. ASIS
8. PSIS
   Follow the iliac crests posteriorly.

9. Sciatic Notch
   Space between the greater trochanter and the ischial tuberosity.

10. Coccyx
    Down the natal cleft

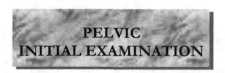

PELVIC INITIAL EXAMINATION

HISTORY:

Patient Name: Date of IE: DX: R/L
Date of onset:
Pain: 0 1 2 3 4 5 6 7 8 9 10   Location:
Current symptoms:

Diagnostic Tests: Meds:

Functional Limitations:
Goals: PMH:

INSPECTION:

RANGE OF MOTION: * = PAIN

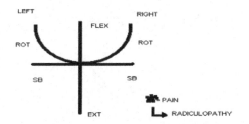

COMMENTS: Flexion:
Extension:
Rotation (ROT):
Sidebend (SB):

MANUAL MUSCLE TEST: 0 – 5/5

Quadriceps: Hamstrings:

Gluteus Medius/Minimus: Hip Adductors:

Tensor Fascia Lata: Gluteus Maximus:

Hip Medial Rotation: Hip Lateral Rotation:

Iliopsoas: Back Extensors:

Abdominals(Rectus):   Trunk Rotaters(Obliques):

MOBILITY TEST: (+) = HYPOMOBILITY   **WNL** = WITHIN NORMAL LIMITS   **(–)** HYPERMOBILITY

Sacroiliac Joint
Posterior – Anterior Glide

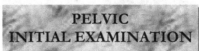

**PELVIC
INITIAL EXAMINATION**

SPECIAL TESTS: * = PAIN

Iliac Compression Test:	(+)	(−)
Iliac Gapping Test:	(+)	(−)
Femoral Nerve Test	(+)	(−)
Hoover Test	(+)	(−)
Straight Leg Raise	(+)	(−)
Sorensen Test	(+)	(−)
Distraction Test	(+)	(−)
Valsalva Maneuver	(+)	(−)
Sitting Flexion Test	(+)	(−)
Standing Flexion Test	(+)	(−)
Stork Test	(+)	(−)
Gillet's Test	(+)	(−)
Leg Length Test	(+)	(−)

                                                      LEFT   RIGHT

(True)   1. Iliac Crest to Greater Trochanter   _____   _____
          2. Greater Trochanter to Lateral knee joint line   _____   _____
          3. Lateral Knee joint line to Medial malleolus   _____   _____

(Apparent/functional)   1. Belly button to Medial malleoli   _____   _____

PALPATION:

OTHER:

ASSESSMENT:

GOALS:

Short Term (0–2 WEEKS)	Long Term (6–8 WEEKS)
1._____	1._____
2._____	2._____
3._____	3._____
4._____	4._____

PLAN: _____ x week for _____ weeks

_____   _____
SIGNATURE   LICENSE #

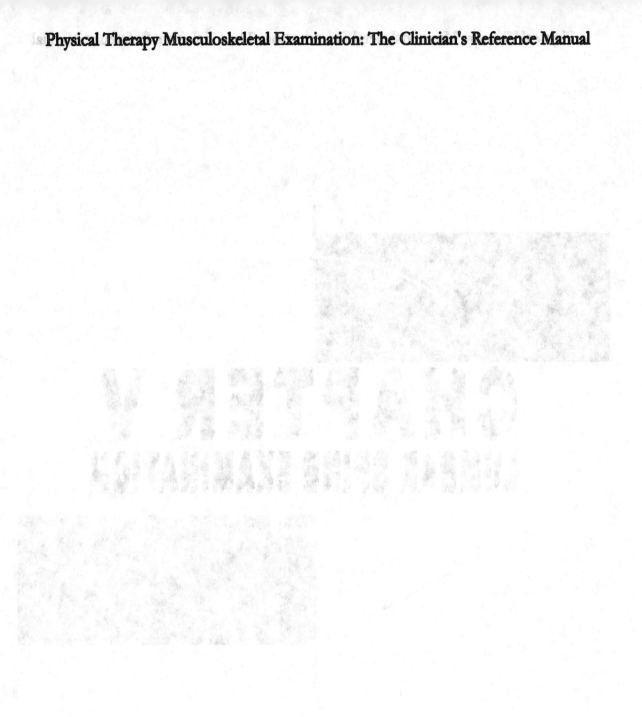

CHAPTER V
LUMBAR SPINE EXAMINATION

NOTES:

I. HISTORY

1. Date of onset of symptoms
2. Mechanism of injury (Traumatic vs. Non-Traumatic)
3. Treatment to date for this injury
4. Current symptoms (Strength, range, edema, pain (0–10 Scale), immobility)
    A. Functional limitations
        a. Home
        b. Work
        c. ADLs

5. Pain (Location, LE radiculopathy, characteristics, intensity, nocturnal)
6. Medications related to injury
7. What makes the symptoms better or worse?
8. Loss of bowel or bladder control
9. Sleep disturbances
10. Diagnostic tests

    A. <u>MRI</u>: (Magnetic Resonance Imaging) Magnetic waves are used to take pictures of slices of the spine. Allows vision of soft tissue, bones, nerves, and disks.
    B. <u>CAT Scan</u>: (Computer Assisted Tomography) X-ray cross sectional views showing the bones of the spine, similar to an MRI.
    C. <u>Myelogram</u>: A test involving placing a dye that shows up on X-ray, into the spinal sac. Will show the places where there is spinal compression.
    D. <u>Discogram</u>: A test where dye is injected directly into the disk at an area of the nucleus pulposus. The dye injection may cause "the pain" or a CAT scan or X-ray will pick up a herniation.
    E. <u>Electromyogram</u>: Looks at the function of the nerve roots leaving the spine. Electrodes placed in the muscles of the lower extremity help identify abnormal nervous signals.
    F. <u>Bone Scan</u>: Helps locate the affected area of the spine. A radioactive chemical is injected into the bloodstream. The chemical attaches itself to areas of bone that are undergoing rapid change. These appear as dark areas on the film.

11. Past medical history
12. Work function
13. Patient's goals

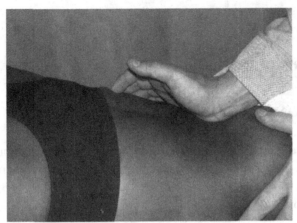

Figure 26

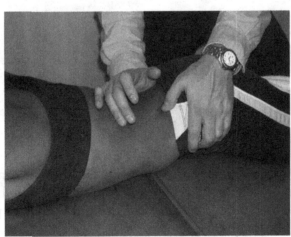

Figure 27

II. INSPECTION

1. Posture (Shift)
2. Atrophy (Standing behind the patient, the clinician looks at the back in extension and flexion)
3. Symmetry of bony landmarks (i.e. Iliac Crests, PSIS, ASIS, Spinous Processes)
4. Swelling
5. Deformities (Scoliosis)
6. Bracing
7. Ability to disrobe

III. LOWER QUARTER SCREEN (See page 3)

IV. RANGE OF MOTION (Lumbar Active-Passive Movements)

Initial pain rating should be established in order to compare movements and pain intensities. Also, the clinician should be in a position to assess the segmental spinal movements. (Patient is standing)

1. Flexion / Extension

2. Sidebending

3. Sidegliding / Translocation

4. Rotation

V. FLEXIBILITY TESTING

1. Hamstrings / Modified Ober's Test / Thomas Test / Ely's Test (See page 29.)

VI. MOBILITY TESTING [3]

1. <u>Posterior-Anterior Glides (Spring Test)</u>: (Patient is supine.) The clinician approximates the **(Figure 26)** spinous process of the vertebra to be mobilized with the ulnar border of the distal hand. The clinician applies an antero-cranial force. A pad may be used to decrease the discomfort at the spinous process.
The clinician assesses: End feel, Muscle guarding, Symmetry, and Motion.

1. <u>Rotational Glide</u>: (Patient is supine.) Standing opposite the mobilizing side, the clinician **(Figure 27)** approximates the transverse process of the vertebra to be mobilized using the ulnar border of the proximal hand. With the distal hand pulling the ASIS posteriorly, the clinician applies an antero-cranial force to the transverse process with the proximal hand. The clinician assesses: End feel, Muscle guarding, Symmetry, and Motion.

NOTES:

VII. MANUAL MUSCLE TESTING [7] (Modified)

1. Back Extensors: (Patient is prone with hands behind the head.) The patient extends through full range.

    A. Grade: 5/5 – Full range and resistance
        4/5 – Same as above, the patient cannot maintain end-range
        3/5 – Completes range with the arms at the sides
        2/5 – Partial range
        1/5 – Palpable contraction

2. Abdominals (Rectus): (Patient is supine with hands behind the head.) The patient curls up, clearing the scapula from the ground.

    A. Grade: 5/5 – Able to come to sitting with back curled
        4/5 – Able to sit with the arms across the chest
        3/5 – Able to sit with the arms outstretched
        2/5 – Unable to complete full motion
        1/5 – Palpable contraction

3. Trunk Rotation(Obliques): (Patient is supine with hands behind the head.) The patient sits up and simultaneously rotates the trunk.

    A. Grade: 5/5 – Full range and hold with hands behind head
        4/5 – Full range with the hands at the sides
        3/5 – Partial range with the hands at the side
        2/5 – Able to approximate the ileum and the ribs
        1/5 – Palpable contraction

Lumbar Spine

NOTES:

VIII. SPECIAL TESTS [1,3]

1. <u>Straight Leg Raise</u> : Nerve tension test. (Patient is supine.) The leg is straightened and raised. Variations include asking the patient simultaneously to raise the head, dorsiflex the foot, and adduct the leg.
    (+) Nerve tension pain around 30° of the leg raise.

2. <u>Hoover Test</u>: Tests for malingering / Wadell Sign. (Patient is supine.) The clinician places one hand under each calcaneous and asks the patient to perform a SLR.
    (+) Clinician feels minimal to no downward force on the opposing foot.

3. <u>Sign of the Buttocks</u>: Tests for a space occupying lesion. (Patient is supine.) The clinician brings the leg into end range hip flexion. The clinician bends the knee to complete further possible range.
    (+) No further range after knee is flexed.

4. <u>Femoral Nerve Stretch</u>: Tests for lesions of the femoral nerve. (Patient is prone) The clinician places the proximal hand superior to the gluteal mass. With the caudal hand, the clinician flexes the knee 90° and extends the hip.
    (+) Provocation of nerve tension pain.

5. <u>Spring Test</u>: Provocation test at the spine. (Patient is prone.) The clinician applies a posterior to anterior mobilization to the lumbar vertebrae using the ulnar aspect of the hand against the spinous process of the vertebra being tested.
    (+) Provocation of the pain.

6. <u>Sorensen Test</u>: Tests lumbar paraspinals. (Patient is prone with trunk in neutral over the edge of table.) The patient is instructed to extend and hold for as long as possible.
    (+) Holding 1 minute or less. (Approximately 3 minutes is normal)

7. <u>Distraction Test</u>: Wadell Sign for the SLR. (Patient is seated.) The knee is brought into extension. (simulating the supine SLR) while the patient is distracted.
    (+) No pain (Patient should experience the same pain as with the SLR)

8. <u>Valsalva Maneuver</u>: Tests intrathecal pressure at the spine. (Patient is seated.) The patient is asked to hold breath and push, as if having a bowel movement.
    (+) Lower back and Sciatic pain.

Lumbar Spine

NOTES:

VIII. SPECIAL TESTS (Continued)

9. <u>Sitting Flexion Test</u>: (Seated position eliminates the effects of the hamstrings.)

> (The patient is seated away from the clinician with the knees flexed 90° resting on a chair.) The clinician maintains both thumbs on either PSIS. The patient is asked to bend forward.
>
> **(+)** Asymmetrical movement of the PSIS indicates **SI** involvement. The side with more cranial motion reveals the side of hypermobility or hypomobility.

10. <u>Standing Flexion Test</u>: (Standing position involves the hamstrings.) (Patient is standing.)

> The clinician maintains thumb position on both PSIS. The patient is asked to bend forward.
>
> **(+)** Asymmetrical movement of the PSIS indicates **IS** involvement. The side with more cranial motion reveals the side of hypermobility or hypomobility.

11. <u>Stork Test</u>: Tests for Pars interarticularis stress fracture / facet involvement.

> (Patient stands on one leg.) The patient is instructed to extend backwards.
>
> **(+)** Pain on the ipsilateral side. (Rotation may be incorporated for facet involvement)
>
> **(+)** Pain on the side of rotation.

12. <u>Iliac Compression Test</u>: Tests for sacroiliac involvement. (Patient is supine.) The clinician crosses hands and places them on either ASIS. The clinician then forces the ileum apart.

> **(+)** Pain at the iliosacral junction posteriorly (Sacroiliac Ligaments).

13. <u>Iliac Gapping Test</u>: Tests for Sacroiliac involvement. (Patient is sidelying.) The clinician pushes down on the iliac crest.

> **(+)** Pain at the iliosacral junction posteriorly.

14. <u>Gillet's Test</u>: Tests for pelvic hypomobility. (Patient is standing.) The clinician maintains thumb position on both PSIS. The patient then brings one knee to chest. The PSIS on the flexed side should drop.

> **(+)** PSIS of the flexing hip moves minimally or remains still.

NOTES:

IX. PALPATION (Symmetry between opposing landmarks)

1. Iliac crests
   Standing and sitting. Look for symmetry.

2. Ischial Tuberosity
   The clinician can find them when the patient is standing with the hip fully flexed or the patient seated / sidelying.
   a. Site of the hamstring origin.

3. Spinous Processes
   Between the iliac crests. Location of L-4

4. Transverse Processes
   On either side of the spinous process. The clinician palpates the ipsilateral process and compresses the contralateral side to feel movement posteriorly.

5. Sacral Sulcus
   Medial gap between the PSIS. Check for symmetrical depth.

6. Pubic Tubercles
   Instruct the patient to palpate the tubercles first. Then, place the hands over the patient's and check for height / pubic symphesis, and anterior / posterior displacement.

7. ASIS

8. PSIS
   Follow the iliac crests posteriorly.

9. Sciatic Notch
   Space between the greater trochanter and the ischial tuberosity.

10. Coccyx
    Down the natal cleft

LUMBAR SPINE
INITIAL EXAMINATION

HISTORY:

Patient Name: Date of IE: DX: R/L

Date of onset:

Pain: 0 1 2 3 4 5 6 7 8 9 10   Location:

Current symptoms:

Diagnostic Tests: Meds:

Functional Limitations:

Goals: PMH:

INSPECTION:

RANGE OF MOTION * = PAIN

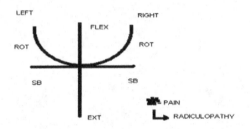

COMMENTS: Flexion:
                       Extension:
                       Rotation (ROT):
                       Sidebend (SB):

MANUAL MUSCLE TEST: 0 – 5/5

Quadriceps:	Hamstrings:
Gluteus Medius/Minimus:	Hip Adductors:
Tensor Fascia Lata:	Gluteus Maximus:
Hip Medial Rotation:	Hip Lateral Rotation:
Iliopsoas:	Back Extensors:
Abdominals(Rectus):	Trunk Rotaters(Obliques):

MOBILITY TEST: (+) = HYPOMOBILITY   **WNL** = WITHIN NORMAL LIMITS   **(–)** = HYPERMOBILITY

Lumbar Zygopophyseal Joints
Posterior – Anterior Glide

LUMBAR SPINE
INITIAL EXAMINATION

SPECIAL TESTS: * = PAIN

Iliac Compression Test:	(+)	(−)
Iliac Gapping Test:	(+)	(−)
Femoral Nerve Test:	(+)	(−)
Hoover Test:	(+)	(−)
Straight Leg Raise:	(+)	(−)
Sorensen Test:	(+)	(−)
Distraction Test:	(+)	(−)
Valsalva Maneuver:	(+)	(−)
Sitting Flexion Test:	(+)	(−)
Standing Flexion Test:	(+)	(−)
Stork Test:	(+)	(−)
Gillet's Test:	(+)	(−)
Leg Length Test:	(+)	(−)

		LEFT	RIGHT
(True)	1. Iliac Crest to Greater Trochanter	_____	_____
	2. Greater Trochanter to Lateral knee joint line	_____	_____
	3. Lateral Knee joint line to Medial malleolus	_____	_____
(Apparent/functional)	1. Belly button to Medial malleoli	_____	_____

PALPATION:

OTHER:

ASSESSMENT:

GOALS:

Short Term (0–2 WEEKS)	Long Term (6–8 WEEKS)
1._____	1._____
2._____	2._____
3._____	3._____
4._____	4._____

PLAN: _____ x week for _____ weeks

_____   _____
SIGNATURE   LICENSE #

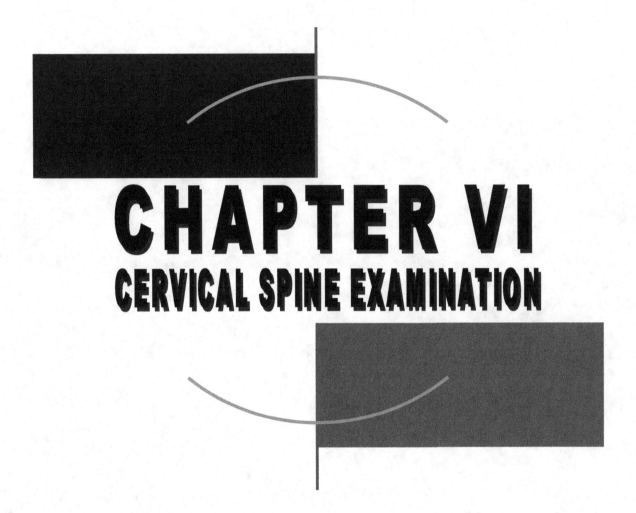

CHAPTER VI
CERVICAL SPINE EXAMINATION

It is important to note that all manual intervention during the assessment and treatment of the cervical spine be preceded by clearing tests including the Vertebral Artery and the Alar Ligament Tests described in this chapter!

NOTES:

I. HISTORY

1. Date of onset of symptoms
2. Mechanism of injury (Traumatic vs. Non-Traumatic)
3. Treatment to date for this injury
4. Current symptoms (Strength, range, edema, pain (0–10 Scale), immobility)
   A. Functional limitations
      a. Home
      b. Work
      c. ADLs

5. Pain (Location, UE radiculopathy, characteristics, intensity, nocturnal)
6. Medications related to injury
7. What makes the symptoms better or worse?
8. Loss of bowel or bladder control
9. Sleep disturbances
10. Diagnostic tests

    A. <u>MRI</u>: (Magnetic Resonance Imaging) Magnetic waves are used to take pictures of slices of the spine. Allows vision of soft tissue, bones, nerves, and disks.
    B. <u>CAT Scan</u>: (Computer Assisted Tomography) X-ray cross sectional views showing the bones of the spine, similar to an MRI.
    C. <u>Myelogram</u>: A test involving placing a dye that shows up on X-ray, into the spinal sac. Will show the places where there is spinal compression.
    D. <u>Discogram</u>: A test where dye is injected directly into the disk at an area of the nucleus pulposus. The dye injection may cause "the pain" or a CAT scan or X-ray will pick up a herniation.
    E. <u>Electromyogram</u>: Looks at the function of the nerve roots leaving the spine. Electrodes placed in the muscles of the lower extremity help identify abnormal nervous signals.
    F. <u>Bone Scan</u>: Helps locate the affected area of the spine. A radioactive chemical is injected into the bloodstream. The chemical attaches itself to areas of bone that are undergoing rapid change. This appear as dark areas on the film.

11. Past medical history
12. Work function
13. Patient's goals

NOTES:

II. INSPECTION

1. Posture (Forward head /rounded shoulders)
2. Atrophy at bilateral shoulder complex
3. Symmetry of bony landmarks
4. Swelling
5. Deformities (Scoliosis)
6. Bracing
7. Ability to disrobe

III. UPPER QUARTER SCREEN (See page 1)

IV. RANGE OF MOTION (Active-Passive Movements)

An initial pain rating should be established in order to compare movements and pain intensities. The clinician should be in a position to assess the spinal movements and end-feel. Measurements can be taken with a tape measure from chin.

1. Flexion / Extension

2. Sidebending

3. Sidegliding / Translocation: (Described in the mobility section)

4. Rotation

V. FLEXABILITY TESTING (Only after screening tests have been completed)

1. <u>Upper Trapezium</u>: (Patient is supine.) The clinician performs an efflurage while holding the patient's head sidebent to the opposite side. Assess trapezium tightness.

2. <u>Scalenes</u>: (Patient is supine with the head in extension.) The clinician palpates just posterior to the sternocleidomastoid.

3. <u>Levator</u>: (Patient is supine.) The clinician fully abducts the patient's arm along the table. If the head moves towards the arm as the arm approaches end range, than it may be restrictive.

4. <u>Pectoralis Minor</u>: Same as the levator, however, the patient's arm will raise off the table.

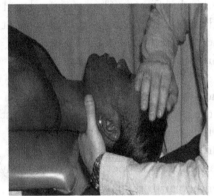
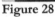

Figure 28

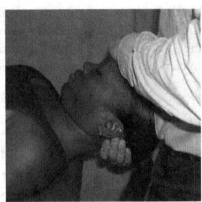

Figure 29

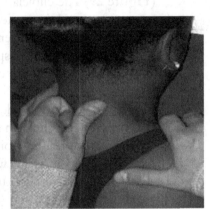

Figure 30

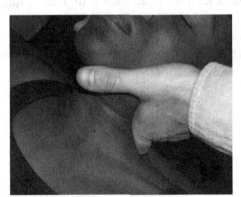

Figure 31

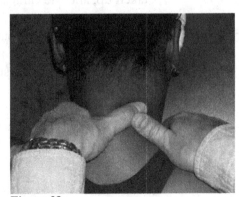

Figure 32

VI. MOBILITY TESTING [3]

1. <u>Distraction Upper Cervical Spine</u>: (Patient is supine at the end of the table in slight extension.) **(Figure 28)** The clinician places the right hand just distal to the occiput at the nuchal line. The neck is cradled in the web space of the thumb and index finger. The opposite hand is placed over the forehead to secure the grip and maintain the angle of extension at the cervical spine. The clinician leans back, applying no more than 5 lbs. of force.

2. <u>Distraction Lower Cervical Spine</u>: (Patient is supine at the end of the table in slight flexion.) **(Figure 29)** The clinician places the right hand just distal to the occiput at the nuchal line. The neck is cradled in the web space of the thumb and index finger. The opposite hand is placed over the forehead to secure the grip and maintain the angle of extension at the cervical spine. The clinician slightly flexes the neck until the nuchal ligament is taught. The clinician leans back, applying no more than 5 lbs. of force.

3. <u>Posterior - Anterior Glide</u>: (Patient is prone with the forehead supported by a pillow.) **(Figure 30)** The clinician approximates the DIP joint line of the thumb against the lateral aspect of the PIP joint of the fully flexed index finger. This forms the "V" shaped hand position for which to mobilize with. The clinician places this hand position against the vertebra to be mobilized and applies a force anterior and superior approximately 45°. For C1 and C2, the force is anterior. (Perpendicular to the table) and for the upper thoracic spin the angle of force is approximately 60° superiorly.

4. <u>Sidegliding</u>: (Patient is supine at the end of the table.) The clinician supports the head from **(Figure 31)** underneath with one hand. With the web space of the thumb and the index finger of the opposite hand, the clinician approximates the lateral aspect of the appropriate segment to be tested. By sidebending the neck over the lateral hand, the slack is taken up, and the clinician applies a lateral force. (Sideglide Left = Right Sidebend)

5. <u>Rotation</u>: (Patient is prone with 2 pillows under the chest and a pillow supporting the forehead.) **(Figure 32)** The clinician places the pad of the thumb lateral to the segment to be rotated and applies an anterior pressure, invoking rotation.

NOTES:

VIII. **MANUAL MUSCLE TESTING**[7] (Capital and Cervical)

1. <u>Neck Flexors</u>: (Patient is supine and asked to tuck the chin to the chest.)
The clinician applies resistance to the forehead.

    A. Grade: 5/5 – Full range and hold against maximal resistance
           4/5 – Full range and hold with moderate resistance
           3/5 – Full range against gravity
           2/5 – Partial range against gravity
           1/5 – Palpable contraction without movement

2. <u>Neck Rotators</u>: (Patient is supine and asked to flex and rotate the head.)
The clinician applies resistance to the lateral forehead.

    A. Grade: 5/5 – Full range and hold against maximal resistance
           4/5 – Full range and hold with moderate resistance
           3/5 – Full range against gravity
           2/5 – Patient rolls head on table without resistance
           1/5 – Palpable contraction without movement

3. <u>Neck Extensors</u>: (Patient is prone and asked to extend the head.)
The clinician applies pressure to the back of the head.

    A. Grade: 5/5 – Full range and hold against maximal resistance
           4/5 – Full range and hold with moderate resistance
           3/5 – Full range against gravity
           2/5 – Partial range against gravity
           1/5 – Palpable contraction without movement

Cervical Spine

NOTES:

IX. SPECIAL TESTS [1,3,5]

1. <u>Vertebral Artery Test</u>: Tests if the vertebral arteries are compromised. (Patient is supine with the eyes open at the edge of the table.) The clinician puts the head into extension and a lateral bend. The clinician then rotates the head to the same side and holds 30 seconds.
(+) Patient feels sick, dizzy, or nastagmus occurs at the eyes.

2. <u>Sharp-Purser Test</u>: Tests instability of C1 on C2. (Patient is seated.) The clinician stabilizes the forehead and applies an anterior pressure to the C2 spinous process. As the patient flexes the head, the clinician applies a posterior force with the palm of the other hand at the forehead.
(+) C2 shifts. This identifies an instability of C1 on C2 and is a red flag to refer back to the M.D.

3. <u>Alar Ligament Stress Test</u>: (Patient is supine.) The clinician stabilizes the C2 spinous process and laminae with a wide pinch grip using the thumb and the index finger. The clinician attempts to side glide the head and C2.
(+) Excessive mobility / possible weak capsular end feel

4. <u>Scalaneus Anticus Test</u>: (Patient is supine or seated.) The clinician applies pressure for 30 seconds at the scalene bellies distally as they insert at the 1st and 2nd ribs. **(+)** Pain provocation at the neck, anterior chest, or intrascapular space.

5. <u>Tinel Signs</u>: (Patient is seated with slight sidebend.) The clinician taps over the C5, C6, C7, C8, T1 spinal roots. **(+)** Pain and tingling throughout the nerve distribution.

6. <u>Brachial Plexus Tension Test</u>: (Patient is supine with the head sidebent away from the testing arm.) The shoulder is abducted and depressed with one hand. The patient's arm is extended at the wrist and flexed at the elbow. The clinician slowly extends the elbow.
(+) Pain, tightness and radicular symptoms

7. <u>Distraction</u>: (Patient is seated.) The clinician places his or her hands bilaterally on the mastoid processes and creates a superior traction force.
(+) Symptoms centralize.

8. <u>Spurling's Test</u>: (Patient is seated.) The clinician sidebends the patient's head and applies a compressive force to the top of the head. Should be done to both sides.
(+) Pain provocation / symptom peripheralization.

9. <u>Adson Maneuver</u>: Tests for thoracic outlet syndrome (Patient is seated with arm in approximately 45° of abduction.) The clinician checks the radial pulse and the patient rotates the head towards the shoulder being tested. The patient then extends the head while the clinician extends and externally rotates the arm. The patient is instructed to take a deep breath.
(+) Pulse disappears.

NOTES:

VIII. SPECIAL TESTS (Continued)

11. <u>Roos Test</u>: Tests for TOS (Patient is seated.) The patient abducts the arms 90° externally rotates the shoulders, flexes the elbows 90°. The arms are horizontally abducted just posterior to the frontal plane. The patient is asked to pump the fists for 3 minutes.
(+) Unable to keep the arms in the starting position, pain, or numbness and tingling.

12. <u>Phalens Test</u>: Test to rule out Carpal Tunnel Syndrome. (Patient is seated.). The patient is asked to press flexed wrists against one another and hold for 1 minute.
(+) Pain at the thenar eminence, 1st, 2nd , and 3rd fingers.

IX. PALPATION

1. Spinous Processes
2. Transverse Processes
    Caudal and anterior to the mastoid processes
3. Articular Pillars
    Inferior and lateral to the C2 spinous process
4. Thyroid cartilage
5. Sternum
6. Clavicle
7. Scapula
8. Hyoid bone
9. Carotid Pulse
10. Mastoid Process
11. C7 / Occiput

CERVICAL SPINE
INITIAL EXAMINATION

HISTORY:

Patient Name: Date of IE: DX: R/L
Date of onset:
Pain: 0 1 2 3 4 5 6 7 8 9 10   Location (Radiculopathy): L / R / B
Current symptoms:

Diagnostic Tests: Meds:

Functional Limitations:
Goals: PMH:

INSPECTION:

RANGE OF MOTION: * = PAIN

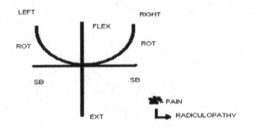

COMMENTS: Flexion:
Extension:
Rotation (ROT):
Sidebend (SB):

MANUAL MUSCLE TEST: 0 – 5/5

Neck Flexors: Neck Extensors:

Neck Rotaters: Shoulder Elevation:

Shoulder Abduction: Elbow Flexion:

Wrist Extension: Elbow Extension:

Wrist Flexion: Thumb Extension:

Finger Adduction:

MOBILITY TEST: (+) = HYPOMOBILITY   **WNL** = WITHIN NORMAL LIMITS   **(–)** = HYPERMOBILITY

Distraction Upper Cervical Spine   Distraction Lower Cervical Spine
Posterior – Anterior Glide   Sidegliding
Rotation

CERVICAL SPINE
INITIAL EXAMINATION

SPECIAL TESTS: * = PAIN

Vertebral Artery Test:	(+)	(−)
Alar Ligament Stress Test:	(+)	(−)
Sharp-Purser Test:	(+)	(−)
Scaleneus Anticus Test:	(+)	(−)
Tinel Sign:	(+)	(−)
Brachial Plexus Tension:	(+)	(−)
Distraction Test	(+)	(−)
Spurling's Test:	(+)	(−)
Adson Maneuver:	(+)	(−)
Roos Test:	(+)	(−)
Phalens Test:	(+)	(−)

PALPATION:

OTHER:

ASSESSMENT:

GOALS:

Short Term (0–2 WEEKS)	Long Term (6–8 WEEKS)
1._____	1._____
2._____	2._____
3._____	3._____
4._____	4._____

PLAN: _____ x week for _____ weeks

_____   _____

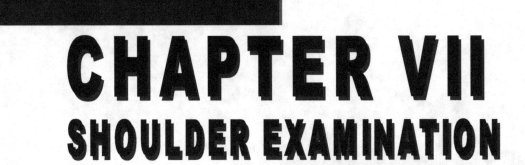

CHAPTER VII
SHOULDER EXAMINATION

NOTES:

I. HISTORY

1. Date of onset of symptoms
2. Mechanism of injury (Traumatic vs. Non-Traumatic)
3. Diagnostic Tests (X-Ray, MRI, Arthrogram)
4. Treatment to date for this injury
5. Current symptoms (Strength, range, edema, pain immobility)
   - A. Functional limitations
     - a. Home
     - b. Work
     - c. ADLs
6. Pain (Location, UE radiculopathy, characteristics, intensity, at night)
7. Medications related to injury
8. Past medical history
9. Work function
10. Patient's goals

II. INSPECTION

1. Atrophy

2. Symmetry

3. Step-Off (AC)

4. Sulcus Sign

5. Scapular position

   A. Winging

   B. Thoracic spine from T2–T7

   C. <u>Sprengel's Deformity</u>: The scapula is abnormally small and out of position.

6. Cervical posture (Forward head / rounded shoulder)

III. UPPER QUARTER SCREEN (See page 1.)

NOTES:

IV. **ACTIVE RANGE OF MOTION**[8] (Look for willingness to move and pain.)

    1. Goniometry (Assess end-feel)

        A. Elevation through the scapular plane and observe scapular rotation.

        B. Appley's Scratch Test
            a. IR behind the back followed by ER over the ipsilateral shoulder.

        C. Horizontal Adduction

        D. Flexion: (Patient is supine.) 0°–180°
                Stationary arm: Midline of the body
                      Apex: Lateral Acromion
                Movement arm: Lateral Epicondyle

        E. Abduction: (Patient is supine.) 0°–180°
                Stationary arm: Midline of the body
                      Apex: Lateral Acromion
                Movement arm: Midline of the Humerus

        F. ER/IR: (Patient is supine.) 0°–90°
                Stationary arm: Perpendicular to the floor
                      Apex: Olecranon Process
                Movement arm: Distal Ulnar Head

        G. Extension: (Patient is prone.)0°–60°
                Stationary arm: Midline of the body
                      Apex: Lateral Acromion
                Movement arm: Lateral Epicondyle

IV. **PASSIVE RANGE OF MOTION** (Same as above)

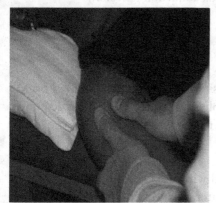

Figure 33

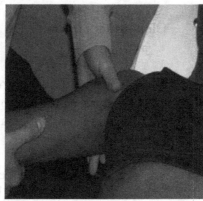

Figure 34

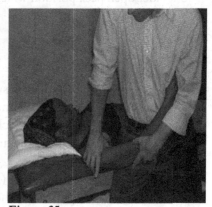

Figure 35

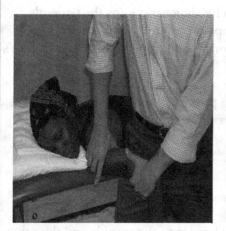

Figure 36

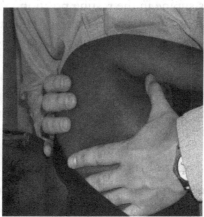

Figure 37

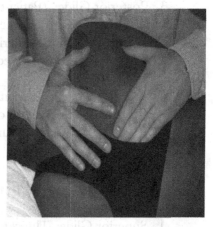

Figure 38

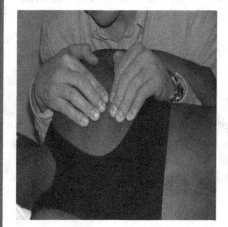

Figure 39A

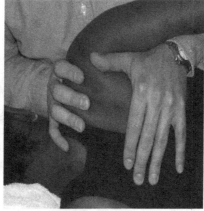

Figure 39B

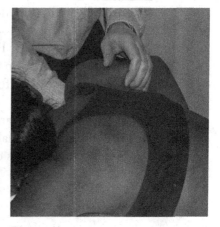

Figure 40

V. MOBILITY TESTING [3]

(Shoulder open pack position which is 55° of abduction and 30° of horizontal adduction / flexion)

Glenohumeral Joint

(Patient is supine.)

1. Distraction: (Patient is supine with the arm in the resting position.) The clinician places both
(Figure 33) hands around the upper arm at the axilla and applies a distractive force by leaning back. The clinician may also grasp just proximal to the wrist and distract the long axis of the arm.

2. Inferior/Caudal Glide: (Patient is in a resting position, seated with the clinician facing the
(Figure 34) patient.) The clinician cups the elbow with the lateral hand and applies an inferior force with the web space of the other hand on the lateral joint line just distal to the acromion.

3. Posterior Glide: (Patient is supine in the resting position.) The clinician clamps the patient's
(Figure 35) hand between the upper arm and ribcage and cups the elbow. With the other hand on the anterior aspect of the shoulder, a posterior force is applied with the clinician's elbow locked out.

4. Anterior Glide: (Patient is prone with the arm in the resting position.) The clinician cups the
(Figure 36) elbow with one hand and applies an anterior force to the posterior aspect of the proximal humerus.

Scapulothoracic Articulation

(Patient is prone or sidelying, facing the clinician.)

1. Superior Glide: The clinician places one hand at the inferior border of the scapula and the other
(Figure 37) on the superior aspect of the acromion and applies a superior force.

2. Inferior Glide: The clinician places one hand at the inferior border of the scapula and the other
(Figure 38) on the superior aspect of the acromion and applies an inferior force.

3. Medial / Lateral Glide: The clinician places one hand at the inferior border of the scapula and
(Figure 39) the other on the superior aspect of the acromion and applies a lateral **(A)** or medial **(B)** force.

4. Distraction: The clinician places the tips of the index through 5th fingers of both hands under the
(Figure 40) infero-medial border of the scapula and distracts the scapula from the ribcage. This technique is easier when performed with the patient is sidelying.

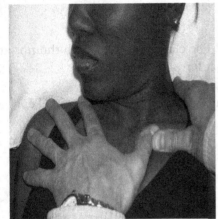

Figure 41

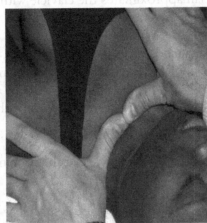

Figure 42

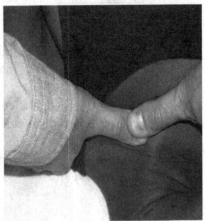

Figure 43

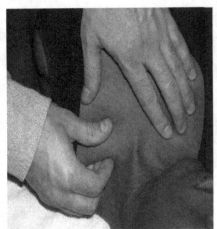

Figure 44

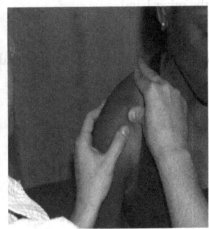

Figure 45

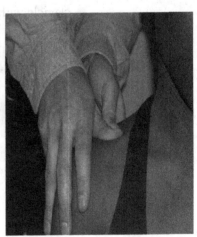

Figure 46

V. MOBILITY TESTING (Continued)

Sternoclavicular Joint

(Patient is supine.)

1. <u>Superior Glide</u>: The clinician approximates the clavicle with both thumbs at the proximal end **(Figure 41)** and provides a supero-medial glide.

2. <u>Inferior Glide</u>: The clinician stands facing the patient's feet. The clinician places both thumbs at **(Figure 42)** the proximal end of the clavicle and provides an infero-lateral glide.

3. <u>Posterior Glide</u>: The clinician approximates the clavicle with both thumbs at the proximal end **(Figure 43)** and provides a posterior glide.

4. <u>Anterior Glide</u>: The clinician gasps the clavicle at the proximal end and pulls anteriorly. **(Figure 44)**

Acromioclavicular Joint

(Patient is seated.)

1. <u>Posterior Glide</u>: The clinician faces the patient and grasps the acromion between the index finger **(Figure 45)** and the thumb with one hand and provides a posterior glide on the distal end of the clavicle with the other hand.

2. <u>Anterior Glide</u>: The clinician faces the back of the patient. The clinician provides an antero- **(Figure 46)** lateral glide, with both thumbs, to the distal end of the clavicle.

NOTES:

VI. MANUAL MUSCLE TESTING (Modified) (Patient goes through full range first.)

1. <u>Resisted Testing:</u> (Done first) Flexion / Extension / ABduction / ADduction
IR/ ER / Elbow Flexion / Elbow Extension / Shrugs

A. <u>Flexion</u>: Tests anterior deltoid, supraspinatus, and corachobrachialis. (Patient is seated.) A break test is performed with the patient's shoulder flexed to 90° with the forearm pronated. The clinician attempts to extend the shoulder at the distal humerus.

B. <u>Scaption</u>: Tests deltoid and supraspinatus. (Patient is seated.) A break test is performed with the patient's shoulder flexed to 90°, horizontally abducted 45° from the midsagital plane, and the forearm is pronated. The clinician attempts to extend and adduct the shoulder at the distal humerus.

C. <u>Abduction</u>: Tests middle deltoid and supraspinatus. (Patient is seated.) A break test is performed with the patient's shoulder abducted to 90° and the forearm pronated. The clinician attempts to adduct the shoulder at the distal humerus.

D. <u>Elbow Flexion</u>: Tests biceps, brachialis, and brachioradialis. (Patient is seated.) A break test is performed in 90° of elbow flexion with the wrist in supination. The clinician attempts to extend the elbow.

E. <u>Horizontal Adduction</u>: Tests pectoralis major. (Patient is supine.) A break test is performed in 90° shoulder flexion and 90° of elbow flexion with the wrist in pronation. The clinician attempts to horizontally abduct the shoulder.

F. <u>Internal Rotation</u>: Tests subscapularis, latissimus, pec major, and teres major. (Patient is prone.)The patient's shoulder is abducted 90°, the elbow is flexed 90° and is hung over the edge of the table. With the patient's head turned to the testing side, a break test is performed with the clinician attempting to externally rotate the shoulder.

G. <u>External Rotation</u>: Tests teres minor and infraspinatus. (The patient is prone.) The patient's shoulder is abducted 90°, the elbow is flexed 90° and is hung over the edge of the table. With the patient's head turned to the testing side, a break test is performed with the clinician attempting to internally rotate the shoulder.

H. <u>Extension</u>: Tests posterior deltoid, lats, and teres major. (Patient is prone.) A Break test is performed with the patient's shoulder extended and the forearm supinated. The clinician attempts to flex the shoulder at the distal humerus.

NOTES:

VI. MANUAL MUSCLE TESTING[7] (Continued)

I. <u>Horizontal Abduction</u>: Tests posterior deltoid. (Patient is prone.) The patient's shoulder is abducted 90°, the elbow is flexed 90° and is hung over the edge of the table. A break test is performed with the clinician attempting to horizontally adduct the shoulder.

J. <u>Elbow Extension</u>: Tests triceps brachii. (Patient is prone.) The patient's shoulder is abducted 90°, the elbow is flexed 90°, the forearm is pronated and hung over the edge of the table. With the distal humerus supported with one hand, a break test is performed in elbow extension. The clinician attempts to flex the elbow.

Scapulothoracic MMT

A. <u>Scapular Abduction and Upward Rotation</u>: Tests serratus anterior. (Patient is seated.) The patient's arm is flexed 130°. With the thumb and index finger, the clinician palpates the infero-lateral border of the scapula, a break test is performed with the clinician's other hand. The clinician attempts to extend the shoulder while palpating activity at the scapula.

B. <u>Scapular Elevation</u>: Tests upper trap. (Patient is seated with hands relaxed in lap.) A break test is performed with the patient attempting to shrug the shoulders. The clinician repeats this on each shoulder, and attempts to pull the shoulders downward.

C. <u>Functional Lats</u>: Tests Lats. (Patient is seated.) With both hands on the table at the patient's side, the patient attempts to clear the buttocks off the table. This motion mimics the function of assisting in transferring.

D. <u>Scapular Adduction</u>: Tests middle fibers of the trap. (Patient is prone.) The patient's shoulder is abducted 90°, the elbow is flexed 90° and is hung over the edge of the table. With one hand the clinician stabilizes the contralateral scapula to prevent rotation. With the testing hand, a break test is performed at the distal humerus. The clinician attempts to push the arm to the floor.

Shoulder

NOTES:

VI. MANUAL MUSCLE TESTING [7] (Continued)

    E. <u>Scapular Depression and Adduction</u>: Tests lower fibers of the trap. (Patient is prone.) The patient's shoulder is abducted 130°, the elbow is extended, and the thumb is pointed toward the ceiling. With one hand the clinician stabilizes the contralateral scapula to prevent rotation. With the testing hand, a break test is performed at the distal humerus. The clinician attempts to push the arm to the floor.

    F. <u>Scapular Adduction and Downward Rotation</u>: Tests rhomboids. (Patient is prone.) The patient is in internal rotation with the arm resting on the lower back. A break test is performed at the distal humerus. The clinician attempts to push the arm downward and outward.

VII. SPECIAL TESTS [1,5]

Anterior Instability

1. <u>Apprehension Test</u>: (Patient is supine with the arm in ER and abducted 90°) The elbow is supported and further ER is **SLOWLY** introduced.
(+) Pain and facial apprehension.

2. <u>Fulcrum Test</u>: Same as the Apprehension Test however, the clinician places a fist underneath the shoulder bringing it anteriorly. ER is **SLOWLY** introduced.
(+) Pain and facial apprehension earlier than the Apprehension Test.

3. <u>Relocation Test or Fowler Sign</u>: Same as the above test however, the clinician applies a posterior force to the glenohumeral joint. ER is **SLOWLY** introduced. (+) Pain and facial apprehension, later in the range than the Apprehension Test

4. <u>Clunk Test</u>: Tests for a labral tear / anterior dislocation. (Patient is supine with the arm fully abducted and externally rotated) The clinician holds this position and with the other hand on the posterior aspect of the humeral head, applies an anterior force.
(+) Pain and clunk sound of humerus over the labrum.

Posterior Instability

5. <u>Push-Pull Test</u>: (Patient is supine.) The clinician holds the patient's arm at the wrist and brings the arm into 90° abduction and 30° flexion. The clinicians' other hand is placed at the anterior aspect of the humeral head. As the patient's wrist is pulled superiorly, a posterior force is applied to the humeral head.
(+) > 50% posterior humeral translation, pain, or apprehension

Shoulder

NOTES:

VII. SPECIAL TESTS (Continued)

6. <u>Posterior Apprehension</u>: (Patient is supine with the arm in 90° scaption and 90° elbow flexion) The clinician applies an axial load to the patient's elbow forcing the humerus posteriorly. Simultaneously, the clinician horizontally adducts and medially rotates the arm.
   (+) Pain and apprehension.

Inferior Instability

7. <u>Sulcus Test</u>: (Patient is sitting with the arm at the side) The clinician pulls the arm inferiorly.
   (+) Thumb widths dimple between the humeral head and the distal acrominon.

Acromioclavicular Joint

(Patient is seated.)

9. <u>Shear Test</u>: The clinician grasps the acromion with one hand and the clavicle with the other hand and applies a posterior and anterior glide.
   (+) Pain, crepitus, and excessive motion.

Muscle / Tendon Pathology

(Patient is seated / standing)

1. <u>Yergason's Test</u>: Tests for long head bicipital tendon subluxation / tendentious.
   (Patient's arm is at the side in 90° elbow flexion and full pronation) The clinician resists the patient attempting to supinate the wrist and externally rotate the shoulder.
   (+) Pain.

2. <u>Speed's Test</u>: Tests for bicipital tendentious. The patient flexes the shoulder to 90° with a straight arm and supinates the wrist. While palpating the bicipital groove, the clinician applies a downward force at the forearm.
   (+) Pain.

3. <u>Drop Arm Test</u>: Tests for a rotator cuff tear. With the arm starting in 90° abduction, the patient is instructed to slowly lower arm to the side. The clinician may apply some eccentric resistance.
   (+) The arm drops quickly and painfully.

4. <u>Empty Can Test</u>: Tests the integrity of the supraspinatus tendon. The patient's arm is placed in abduction and the clinician applies resistance. The arm is then placed in 90° of scaption and full IR. Resistance is again applied.
   (+) Pain, weakness, and inability to hold resistance.

NOTES:

VII. SPECIAL TESTS (Continued)

5. <u>Neer Impingement Test</u>: Tests for supraspinatus impingement. The clinician forces end range shoulder flexion approximating the greater tuberosity and the antero-inferior aspect of the underside of the acromion.
   (+) Pain.

6. <u>Hawkins-Kennedy Impingement Test</u>: Tests for supraspinatus impingement. The patient's shoulder is in full IR, flexed 90° with the elbow flexed 90°. The clinician holds the patient's arm at the elbow and forces shoulder HADD with IR.
   (+) is Pain.

7. <u>Lift off Test</u>: Tests for a subscapularis tear. The patient's elbow is flexed and the shoulder is internally rotated behind the back. Maintaining this position, the patient is asked to lift the hand from the back.
   (+) Pain and inability to lift.

VII. PALPATION

1. Suprasternal notch
2. SC Joint
3. Clavicle
4. Coracoid Process
5. AC Joint
6. Acromion and borders
7. Greater Tuberosity (IR arm)
8. Bicipital Groove
9. Lesser Tuberosity
10. Scapula
    A. Spine
    B. Vertebral / Lateral borders
    C. Superior / Inferior angles
11. Sternocleidomastoid
12. Pectoralis Major and insertion
13. Biceps
14. Deltoid
15. Trapezium
16. Supraspinatus Belly and Tendon (At the greater tuberosity with the arm in IR behind back)
17. Infraspinatus Belly and Tendon
    A. (At the postero-lateral corner of the acromion with the arm behind the back)
18. Teres Minor (Arm externally rotated)
19. Latissimus Dorsi
20. Serratus Anterior (Arm is in an extended, punch position)
21. Axillary borders
22. Subacromial Bursa (With the arm in extension)

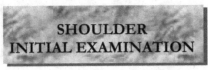

SHOULDER
INITIAL EXAMINATION

HISTORY:

Patient Name: Date of IE: DX: R/L

Date of onset:

Pain: 0 1 2 3 4 5 6 7 8 9 10   Location:

Current symptoms:

Diagnostic Tests: Meds:

Functional Limitations:

Goals: PMH:

INSPECTION:

RANGE OF MOTION * = PAIN

Flexion: _____   Abduction: _____   Extension: _____   IR: _____   ER: _____

MANUAL MUSCLE TEST: 0 – 5/5

Flexion:	Scaption:
Abduction:	Horizontal Adduction:
Elbow Flexion:	Elbow Extension:
Internal Rotation:	External Rotation:
Extension:	Horizontal Abduction:
Scapular Abduction and Upward Rotation:	Scapular Adduction:
Scapular Elevation:	Functional Lats:
Scapular Depression and Adduction:	Scapular Adduction and Downward Rotation:

MOBILITY TEST: **(+)** = HYPOMOBILITY   **WNL** = WITHIN NORMAL LIMITS   **(−)** = HYPERMOBILITY

Glenohumeral Joint
Anterior Glide
Posterior Glide
Distraction
Inferior / Caudal Glide

Sternoclavicular Joint
Anterior Glide
Posterior Glide
Superior Glide

Scapulothoracic Articulation
Distraction
Superior Glide
Inferior Glide
Medial / Lateral Glide

Acromioclavicular Joint
Anterior Glide
Posterior Glide
Inferior Glide

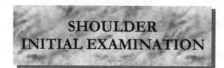

**SHOULDER
INITIAL EXAMINATION**

SPECIAL TESTS: * = PAIN

Anterior Instability

Apprehension Test:	(+) (–)
Fulcrum Test:	(+) (–)
Relocation Test:	(+) (–)
Clunk Test:	(+) (–)
Push – Pull Test:	(+) (–)

Posterior Instability

Push – Pull Test:	(+) (–)
Posterior Apprehension:	(+) (–)

Inferior Instability

Sulcus Sign:	(+) (–)

Muscle Tendon Pathology

Yergason's Test:	(+) (–)
Speed's Test:	(+) (–)
Drop Arm:	(+) (–)
Empty Can Test:	(+) (–)
Hawkins-Kennedy Test:	(+) (–)
Neer Impingement Test:	(+) (–)
Lift Off Test:	(+) (–)

Acromioclavicular Joint

Shear Test:	(+) (–)

PALPATION:

OTHER: (Girth)

ASSESSMENT:

GOALS:

Short Term (0–2 WEEKS)	Long Term (6–8 WEEKS)
1._____	1._____
2._____	2._____
3._____	3._____
4._____	4._____

PLAN: _____ x week for _____ weeks

_____   _____
SIGNATURE   LICENSE #

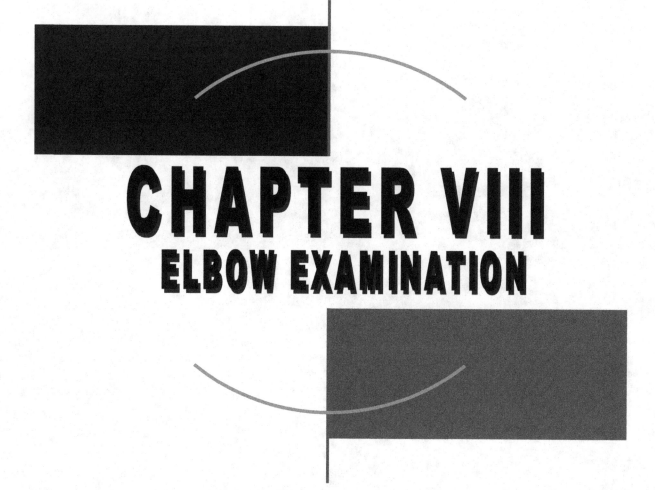

CHAPTER VIII
ELBOW EXAMINATION

Elbow

NOTES:

I. HISTORY

1. Date of onset of symptoms
2. Mechanism of injury (Traumatic vs. Non-Traumatic)
3. Diagnostic tests (X-Ray, MRI, Arthrogram)
4. Treatment to date for this injury
5. Current symptoms (Strength, range, edema, pain immobility)
   A. Functional limitations
      a. Home
      b. Work
      c. ADLs
6. Pain (Location, characteristics, intensity, at night)
7. Medications related to injury
8. Past medical history
9. Patient's goals

II. INSPECTION

1. Muscle atrophy / hypertrophy
2. Symmetry
3. Shoulder height
4. Carrying angle in standing
5. Amount of resting flexion at the elbow
6. Wrist function
7. Unusual swelling at the common flexor / extensor tendon insertions
8. Injection site, if reported in the patient history

III. UPPER QUARTER SCREEN (See page 1)

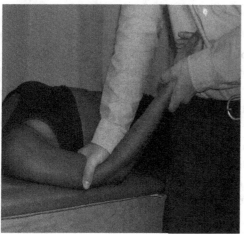

Figure 47

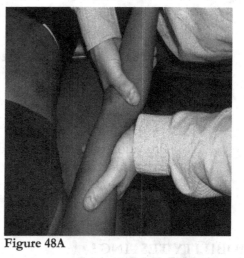

Figure 48A

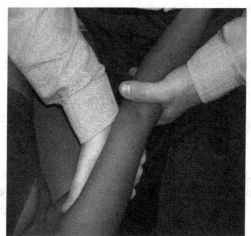

Figure 48B

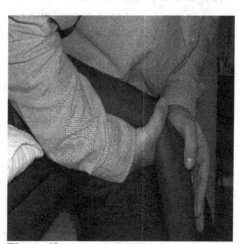

Figure 49

IV. RANGE OF MOTION [8]

1. Goniometry (Assess end-feel)

    A. Extension / Flexion: (Patient is supine.) 0° – 140°
          Stationary arm: Lateral midline of the humerus
          Movement arm: Lateral midline of the radius (Radial head/Radial styloid process)
          Apex: Lateral epicondyle of the humerus

    A. Supination: (Patient is seated with 90° elbow flexion) 0° – 80°
          Stationary arm: Parallel to the anterior midline of the humerus
          Movement arm: Across ventral aspect of the wrist, proximal to the styloid processes
          Apex: Medial to the ulnar styloid process

    B. Pronation: (Patient is seated with 90° elbow flexion) 0° – 80°
          Stationary arm: Parallel to the anterior midline of the humerus
          Movement arm: Across dorsal aspect of the wrist, proximal to the styloid processes
          Apex: Lateral to the ulnar styloid process

V. MOBILITY TESTING [3]

Humeroulnar Joint

1. <u>Distraction</u>: (Patient is supine with the elbow flexed 90° and the forearm supinated) The **(Figure 47)** clinician grasps the back of the supinated wrist with one hand and stabilizes the humerus against the table with the other hand. The clinician pulls the ulna upwards perpendicular to the humerus.

2. <u>Medial - Lateral Glide</u>: (Patient is supine with the elbow in slight flexion) The clinician grasps **(Figure 48)** and stabilizes the proximal forearm with one hand. With the other hand, the clinician grasps the humeral epicondyle. If this hand is on the medial aspect of the joint, then a lateral glide is performed **(A)** and if it is at the lateral aspect, then a medial glide is performed. **(B)**

3. <u>Anterior Glide</u>: (Patient is prone with the shoulder abducted 90° and fully internally rotated, **(Figure 49)** rested on the clinician's thigh) The clinician stabilizes the distal humerus with the medial hand. With the heel of the lateral hand, an anterior force is applied to the olecranon process (along the shaft of the ulna).

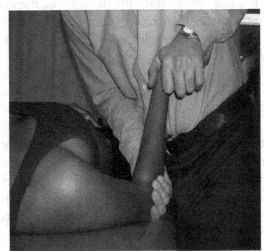

Figure 50

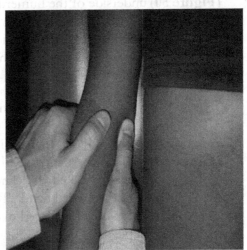

Figure 51

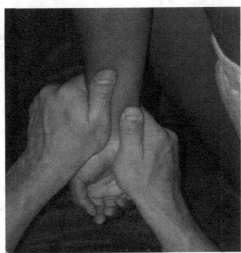

Figure 52

V. MOBILITY TESTING [3] (Continued)

Humeroradial Joint

1. <u>Approximation</u>: (Patient is supine with the elbow flexed 90°) The clinician stabilizes the
(Figure 50) underside of the humerus with the proximal hand. With the distal hand, the clinician approximates the thenar eminence to thenar eminence of the patient with the patient's wrist in extension. A downward force through the wrist along the axis of the radius is applied. This technique can be combined with supination and pronation.

Proximal Radioulnar Joint

1. <u>Anterior - Posterior Glide</u>: (Patient is supine with the arm at the side and the elbow slightly
(Figure 51) flexed. The patient, with the wrist in neutral gently grasps the clinicians medial aspect of the elbow. The clinician stabilizes the distal humerus and proximal radius with the medial hand. The thumb is placed over the anterior radial head and the index finger is placed over the posterior aspect. An anterior and posterior force is applied.

Distal Radioulnar Joint

1. <u>Anterior – Posterior Glide</u>: (Patient is supine or seated with the elbow bent and the wrist in
(Figure 52) neutral) With one hand the clinician stabilizes the radius between the heel of the hand and the index through 5th finger. With the other hand, the clinician grasps the distal ulna and glides in an anterior or posterior manner.

VI. FLEXIBILITY TESTING

1. <u>Wrist Extensor Flexibility</u>: (Patient is seated.) The patient's elbow is fully extended and pronated with the shoulder in slight flexion. The wrist is moved into flexion and ulnar deviation.

2. <u>Wrist Flexor Flexibility</u>: (Patient is seated.) The patient's elbow is extended and supinated with the shoulder in slight flexion. The wrist is moved into extension.

Elbow

NOTES:

VII. MANUAL MUSCLE TEST [7] (Bilaterally)

1. Biceps Brachii: (Patient is seated.) A break test is performed in flexion with the wrist in supination. The clinician attempts to extend the elbow.

2. Brachialis: (Patient seated.) A break test is performed in flexion with the wrist in pronation. The clinician attempts to extend the elbow.

3. Brachioradialis: (Patient is seated.) A break test is performed in flexion with the wrist midway between supination and pronation. The clinician attempts to extend the elbow.

4. Triceps Brachii: (Patient is prone with the shoulder 90° abducted.) A break test is performed in extension. The clinician attempts to flex the elbow.

5. Supinator: (Patient is seated with the arm at the side and the elbow flexed 90°. The wrist is in mid-position) A break test is performed with the clinician attempting to pronate the forearm.

6. Pronator Teres / Quadratus: (Patient is seated with the arm at the side and the elbow flexed 90°. The wrist is in mid-position) A break test is performed with the clinician attempting to supinate the forearm.

7. Flexor Carpi Radialis: (Patient is seated.) A break test is performed with the wrist in flexion. The clinician attempts to extend and ulnar deviate the wrist. Pressure is applied over the second metacarpal.

8. Flexor Carpi Ulnaris: (Patient is seated.) A break test is performed with the wrist in flexion. The clinician attempts to extend and radial deviate the wrist. Pressure is applied over the fifth metacarpal.

9. Extensor Carpi /Radialis Brevis, Longus, Ulnaris: (Patient is seated.) A break test is performed with the wrist in extension. The clinician attempts to flex the wrist.

10. Finger Extension: (Patient is seated with the wrist in pronation. The MCP and IP joints are in relaxed flexion.) With pressure just distal to all MCP joints, a break test is performed with the clinician attempting to flex the digits.

11. Grip Strength: (Patient is seated with the arm at the side and the elbow flexed 90°) A Grip dynamometer is used. Three trials attempted by patient bilaterally. Non-dominant hand should be no less than 5% –10% of the dominant hand[1].

NOTES:

VIII. SPECIAL TESTS [1,3,5]

1. <u>Valgus Stress Test</u>: (Patient is seated and the test is repeated with the elbow in slight flexion, 90° flexion, and full flexion) With the proximal hand, the clinician stabilizes the humerus and with the distal hand, the clinician secures just above the wrist. While palpating the ulnar collateral ligament, the clinician applies a valgus / medial force to the distal forearm.
   (+) Pain or hypermobility at:

> Slight flexion: Anterior Bundle
> 90° flexion: Transverse Bundle
> Full Flexion: Posterior Bundle

2. <u>Varus Stress Test</u>: (Patient is seated and the test is repeated with the elbow in slight flexion, 90° flexion, and full flexion) With the proximal hand, the clinician stabilizes the humerus and with the distal hand the clinician secures just above the wrist. While palpating the radial collateral ligament, the clinician applies a varus / lateral force to the distal forearm.
   (+) Pain or hypermobility at:

> Slight flexion: Anterior Band
> 90° flexion: Medial Band
> Full Flexion: Posterior Band

3. <u>Cozen's Test</u>: Tests for lateral epicondylitis. The clinician's proximal hand stabilizes the elbow with the thumb palpating the lateral epicondyle. The patient is asked to make a fist, fully pronate the forearm, and extend and radially deviate the wrist. The clinician applies pressure in the opposite of these directions.
   (+) Lateral epicondyle pain

4. <u>Mill's Test</u>: Tests for lateral epicondylitis. The clinician pronates the forearm, brings the wrist into full flexion and extends the elbow while palpating the lateral epicondyle.
   (+) Lateral epicondyle pain

5. <u>Medial Epicondylitis Test</u>: Tests for medial epicondylitis. The clinician supinates the forearm, brings the wrist into full extension and extends the elbow while palpating the medial epicondyle.
   (+) Medial epicondyle pain.

6. <u>Pronator Teres Syndrome Test</u>: (Patient is seated with forearm supinated and elbow flexed 90°) The clinician resists pronation and elbow extension.
   (+) Numbness and tingling at the median nerve distribution.

NOTES:

VIII. SPECIAL TESTS (Continued)

7. <u>Wartenberg's Sign</u>: (Patient sits with his or her hand resting on table and the fingers passively spread apart) The clinician asks the patient to squeeze the fingers together.
   (+) Inability to approximate 5th digit: ulnar neuropathy.

8. <u>Tinel's Sign</u>: Tests for ulnar nerve involvement. The clinician taps over the ulnar nerve between the olecranon process and the medial epicondyle.
   (+) Tingling at the ulnar distribution distal to the test site.

9. <u>Phalens Test</u>: Tests for carpal Tunnel Syndrome. (Patient is seated.). The patient is asked to press flexed wrists against one another and hold for 1 minute.
   (+) Pain at the thenar eminence, 1st, 2nd , and 3rd fingers.

IX. PALPATION

1. Cubital Fossa
2. Pronator Teres (Medially)
3. Brachioradialis (Laterally)
4. Biceps tendon
5. Brachial Artery
6. Radial Head
7. Coronoid Process of the ulna
8. Medial Epicondyle
       Common insertion for wrist flexors
9. Lateral Epicondyle
       Common insertion for the wrist extensors
10. Medial collateral Ligament
11. Lateral Collateral Ligament
12. Annular Ligament(Proximal to radial head)
13. Olecranon Process (Elbow flexed to 90°)
14. Olecranon Bursa
15. Triceps insertion and muscle belly
12. Biceps insertion and muscle belly

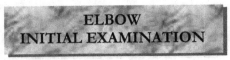

ELBOW
INITIAL EXAMINATION

HISTORY:

Patient Name: Date of IE: DX: R/L

Date of onset:

Pain: 0 1 2 3 4 5 6 7 8 9 10   Location:

Current symptoms:

Diagnostic Tests: Meds:

Functional Limitations:

Goals: PMH:

INSPECTION:

RANGE OF MOTION: * = PAIN

Extension - Flexion: _____   Supination: _____   Pronation: _____

MANUAL MUSCLE TEST: 0 – 5/5

Biceps Brachii: Brachialis:

Pronator Teres / Quadratus: Flexor Carpi Radialis:

Flexor Carpi Ulnaris: Extensor Carpi /Radialis Brevis, Longus, Ulnaris:

Finger Extension: Grip Strength:

MOBILITY TEST: (+) = HYPOMOBILITY   **WNL** = WITHIN NORMAL LIMITS   **(−)** = HYPERMOBILITY

Humeroulnar Joint   **Humeroradial Joint**
Distraction   Approximation
Medial – Lateral Glide
Anterior Glide

Proximal Radioulnar Joint   **Distal Radioulnar Joint**
Antero-Posterior Glide   Antero-Posterior Glide

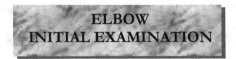

**ELBOW
INITIAL EXAMINATION**

SPECIAL TESTS: * = PAIN

Valgus Stress Test:	(+) (−)
Varus Stress Test:	(+) (−)
Cozen's Test:	(+) (−)
Mill's Test:	(+) (−)
Medial Epicondylitis Test:	(+) (−)
Pronator Teres Syndrome Test:	(+) (−)
Wartenberg's Sign:	(+) (−)
Tinel's Sign:	(+) (−)
Phalens Test:	(+) (−)

PALPATION:

OTHER: (Girth)

ASSESSMENT:

GOALS:

Short Term (0–2 WEEKS)	Long Term (6–8 WEEKS)
1._____	1._____
2._____	2._____
3._____	3._____
4._____	4._____

PLAN: ____ x week for _____ weeks

_____   _____
SIGNATURE   LICENSE #

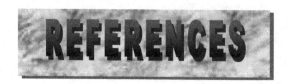

1. Magee, David J. *Orthopedic Physical Assessment, Third Edition.* Philadelphia. W.B. Saunders Company, 1997.

2. Guide To Physical Therapy Practice. *Physical Therapy.* 1997;77: 1629–1631.

3. Hertling, Darlene and Kessler, Randolph M. *Management of Common Musculoskeletal Disorders, Physical Therapy Principles and Methods.* Lipincott, 1996.

4. Skinner, B. Harry. *Current Diagnosis and Treatment in Orthopedics.* Appleton and Lange, 1995.

5. Rothstein, Jules M., Roy, Serge H., Wolw, Steven L. *The Rehabilitation Specialist Handbook, Second Edition.* Philadelphia. F.A. Davis Company, 1998.

6. Hayes, Karen W. *Manual for Physical Agents, Fourth Edition.* Norwalk. Appleton and Lange, 1993.

7. Hislop, Helen J. and Montgomery, Jacqueline. *Daniels and Worthingham's Muscle Testing: Techniques of Manual Examination.* 6th Edition. Philadelphia. W.B. Saunders Company, 1995

8. Norkin, Cynthia C. and White, D. Joyce. *Measurement of Joint Motion: A Guide to Goniometry.* Philadelphia. F.A. Davis Company, 1995.

9. O'Sullivan, Susan B. and Schmitz, Thomas J. *Physical Rehabilitation: Assessment and Treatment.* 3rd Edition. Philadelphia, F.A. Davis Company, 1994.

10. Norkin, Cynthia C. and Levangie, Pamela K. *JointStructure and Function: A Comprehensive Analysis.* 2nd Edition. Philadelphia. F.A. Davis Company, 1992.

11. Kisner, Carolyn and Colby, Lynn Allen. *Therapeutic Exercise Foundations and Techniques.* 3rd Edition. Philadelphia. F.A. Davis Company, 1996.

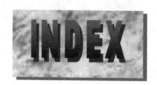

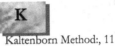

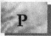

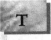

FIGURE INDEX